THE TV VET DOG BOOK

To my good friend

PHILIP WOOD

whose energy, skill

and enthusiasm

have contributed so much

to the success of the

TV Vet Book Series

THE TV VET DOG BOOK

Recognition and Treatment of Common Dog Ailments

By
THE TV VET

FARMING PRESS LIMITED
WHARFEDALE ROAD IPSWICH SUFFOLK

FIRST PUBLISHED 1974

SECOND (REVISED) EDITION 1978

THIRD (REVISED) EDITION 1980

ISBN 0 85236 105 X

Printed in England by
Page Bros (Norwich) Ltd.

Contents

PARASITIC DISEASES

VIRUS DISEASES

GENERAL DISEASES AND CONDITIONS

ACKNOWLEDGEMENTS

We acknowledge with thanks permission to reproduce the following illustrations:
Vertical section of the ear—page 193 (from *Canine Medicine,* 1st Catcott edition, p. 732, American Veterinary Publications, Inc.).
Most common sites for urinary calculi—page 176 (from *Urolithiasis,* Client Education Series, Elanco Products Ltd).
Normal anatomy of hip joint and moderate and advanced dysplasia—pages 107–108 (from *The Disjointed Hip,* Client Education Series, Elanco Products Ltd). Anatomy of Dog—page 14 (from *Canine Anatomy: Organs and Skeleton,* Client Education Series, Elanco Products Ltd).
The outer surface of two minute lobules of the lung—page 132 (from *Black's Veterinary Dictionary,* 10th edition, edited by W C. Miller and G. P. West, A. and C. Black Ltd).
Cross-section of a dog's tooth—page 179 (from *Pedigree Digest,* Vol. 1, No. 1, Autumn/Winter 1973, Pedigree Petfoods Ltd).
Dog flea—page 78 (from *Veterinary Parasitology,* 2nd edition, fig. 346. Oliver and Boyd, by permission of Dr. F. G. A. M. Smith, Dept. of Entomology, British Museum—Natural History).
Dog Louse—page 79 (from *Mem. Pacific Coast Entomol. Soc.* G. F. Ferris 1951 page 236, figure 103).
Bulbous urethra—page 60; Skull of a dog—page 129; heart of a dog, left side—page 138; larynx—page 122; the dog's dentition—page 178; (from *The Anatomy of the Domestic Animal,* by Sisson and Grossman, 4th edition, W. B. Saunders Company of Philadelphia and London).

Foreword

By **JAMES HERRIOT**
Author of "If Only They Could Talk", "It Shouldn't Happen to a Vet",
"Let Sleeping Vets Lie", "Vet in Harness" and
the American edition, "All Creatures Great and Small".

WHY DO dogs have such a claim on our affections? Why do they have the power to cheer or depress us and why does their neglect fill us with such repugnance?

I have thought a lot about this and I feel there is more to it than the fact that they dispense friendliness and love freely and without question. I think the main reason is their utter dependence. They rely on us completely. In our hands lies the capacity to make their lives happy or miserable, and only the dedicated owner knows the boundless satisfaction which comes from conferring pleasure and contentment on his pet, be it pedigree or mongrel.

But caring is not enough. It must be combined with knowledge and here within the pages of this book the knowledge is available to us, simply and attractively presented.

The TV Vet is my lifelong and cherished friend. In writing his book he draws on more than three decades of practical experience and his findings, opinions and advice are gleaned not from others but from the things he has seen, the things he has done. And, just as important, he is a dog lover, deeply involved with and attached to his own animals. The compassion which is a part of him has illumined his professional life and shines through his writing. I can think of no person better equipped to produce a book on the care of dogs.

In the course of my own work many people say to me, "I'd like to have been a vet". There must be millions of frustrated animal doctors around and this is the book for them. It will not make them into veterinary surgeons but it will enable them to take an intelligent interest in their pets and will provide an insight into their ailments. As always, The TV Vet writes with an incisive clarity which cuts through the verbiage of the average text book, and his easily understood descriptions are admirably backed by the excellent illustrations.

I give this book my wholehearted blessing. I hope it will be read and read again by countless people, because I am convinced that the result will be many happier owners, many happier dogs.

James Herriot

Author's Preface

AGAIN AND AGAIN through the years I have been asked the same set of questions by puzzled dog clients. This book attempts to answer all the queries in a simple straightforward manner.

It is my one regret that economics have prevented the use of coloured illustrations. However, my photographer, Tony Boydon, and I have done our utmost with black and white, even though we have found dogs much more difficult to photograph than horses, cattle, sheep or pigs.

The text comes from hard-earned experience in thirty-four years of general practice. During that time I have witnessed with great satisfaction, pleasure and just a little pride the ever-improving canine surgical and medicinal techniques. There can be no doubt that the modern British dog now gets just as good and, in many instances, much better attention and treatment than do most humans.

This book is aimed at providing dog owners with a genuine understanding of their pet's potential illnesses so that the owners can co-operate to the full with the veterinary profession in the prevention and early treatment of disease. At the same time it should serve as a reference book for veterinary students and young graduates.

In addition to my photographer, Tony Boydon, who took all the pictures, I would like to thank Richard Perry who drew the diagrams and all the members of my staff who helped in any way.

GENERAL ADVICE

ANATOMY OF THE DOG

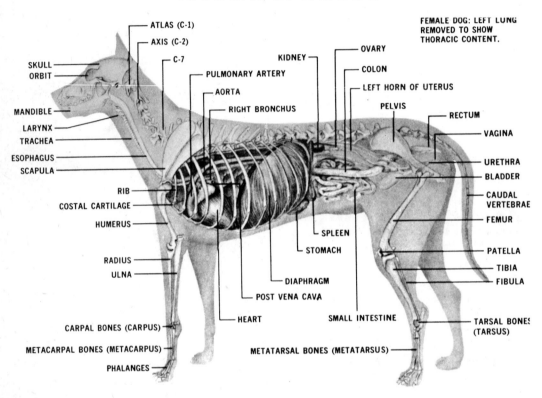

ATLAS (C-1)

AXIS (C-2)

C-7

SKULL

ORBIT

KIDNEY

PULMONARY ARTERY

MANDIBLE

LARYNX

TRACHEA

ESOPHAGUS

SCAPULA

RIB

COSTAL CARTILAGE

HUMERUS

RADIUS

ULNA

AORTA

RIGHT BRONCHUS

OVARY

COLON

LEFT HORN OF UTERUS

PELVIS

RECTUM

VAGINA

URETHRA

BLADDER

CAUDAL VERTEBRAE

FEMUR

PATELLA

TIBIA

FIBULA

SPLEEN

STOMACH

DIAPHRAGM

POST VENA CAVA

HEART

SMALL INTESTINE

TARSAL BONES (TARSUS)

CARPAL BONES (CARPUS)

METACARPAL BONES (METACARPUS)

PHALANGES

METATARSAL BONES (METATARSUS)

FEMALE DOG: LEFT LUNG REMOVED TO SHOW THORACIC CONTENT.

14

1
Feeding

INCORRECT FEEDING not only pre-disposes to obesity *(photo 1)* but is a common cause of skin troubles, hysteria, muscular dystrophy (wasting of the muscles) and other disorders.

The simple fact to bear in mind continu-ally is that dogs are carnivores, i.e. meat-eating animals *(photo 2)*. In their natural state they would eat only raw meat and bones with an occasional mouthful of wild herbs or grasses to supply essential vita-mins and minerals.

Obviously, therefore, the ideal way to keep your dog dietetically healthy is to

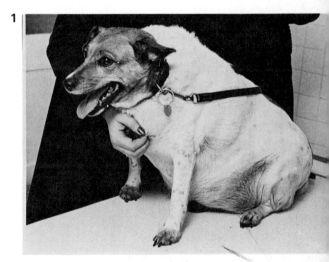
1

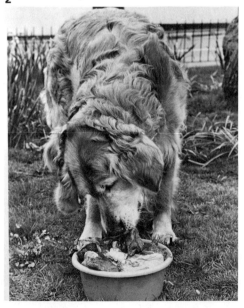
2

stick to the natural diet and feed only raw meat with a small quantity of raw green vegetables mixed in with it *(photo 3)*. A

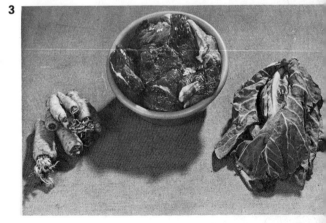
3

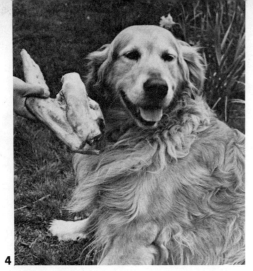
4

large raw bone may be provided once a week *(photo 4)* but all small bones should be avoided, e.g. chop bones, small vertebrae, etc. The modern domesticated dog tends to swallow the occasional small bone whole and this produces an obstruction of the oesophagus or intestine with all the resultant worries and complications of surgical removal.

So-called 'dog chews' are equally dangerous, in fact more so because there is some evidence that they predispose to the formation of urinary calculi (stones in the kidneys, ureters, bladder and urethra).

Satisfactory protein substitutes for meat are eggs, cheese, fish and white meat (chicken and rabbit, etc) but again all fish, poultry and rodent bones must be rigorously withheld.

Dog biscuits and meal should be kept in reserve and *used only when the correct protein foodstuffs are unobtainable,* though **5** with most of the larger breeds a percentage

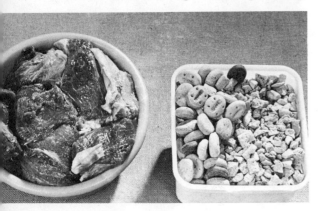

may have to be used to make up sufficient bulk *(photo 5)*.

An ideal diet, therefore, would be as follows:

FIRST CATEGORY—*Puppies from Weaning to 10 Weeks of Age*
Four feeds daily varying in quantity according to breed and size.

1st feed 8 a.m.	A raw or finely chopped hard boiled egg.
2nd feed 1 p.m.	Cheese grated with finely shred raw lettuce, carrots, cabbage or cauliflower.
3rd feed 6 p.m.	Raw red meat—minced. Also containing shreds of raw green vegetables.
4th feed 10–11 p.m.	Raw or cooked red or white meat again with added green vegetables.
For drinking	Both milk and water with the water available ad lib.

So far as quantities are concerned, the smaller breeds should have a total daily bulk of at least 4 oz (113 g) and the larger breeds at least one pound.

SECOND CATEGORY—*From 10 to 16 weeks of age (photo 6)*
The quantities should be gradually increased as the dog grows: the basic foodstuffs should be kept the same but milk can be cut out and water only provided: the number of feeds should be reduced to three per day—8 a.m., 2 p.m. and 8 p.m.

To offset expense, up to 10 per cent of biscuits or meal may be added to the daily bulk which should at 16 weeks have risen to 8 oz (226 g) for the smaller breeds and 2 lb (0·908 kg) for the large.

THIRD CATEGORY—*After 16 Weeks*
Two feeds a day should be given—at 8 a.m. and 8 p.m.—and this twice daily feeding should be continued for the remainder of

16

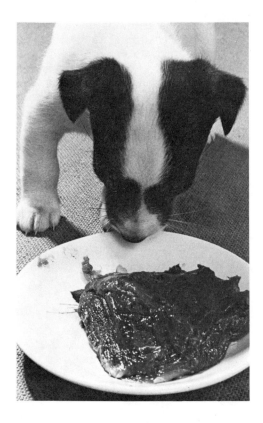

Compound Foods

Synthetic meat made from soya and other high protein vegetables provides an ideal dog food, but unfortunately this is not yet generally available in this country.

Compound meal mixtures can produce a satisfactory feed for a time but their continued use predisposes to eczematous skin and ear eruptions.

Obviously, therefore, in the interests of sensible economy each owner has to compromise, using as much of the ideal foods as possible and padding out with the substitutes.

Quantities

The dog is not a fully grown adult until it is nine months old. Quantities therefore should be gradually increased from four months onwards.

The average sized adult small dog

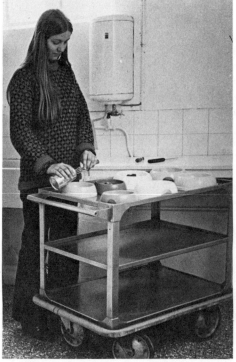

7

the dog's life. In my opinion, the fashionable once daily feeding of adult dogs is unkind and predisposes to scavenging which can result in the swallowing of stones or other foreign bodies.

Canned Dog Foods

Most canned dog foods have added vitamins and minerals and make an excellent feed but it is vital to bear in mind that the canned meats often contain a high percentage of water (up to 87 per cent in some cases) *(photo 7)*. Obviously, therefore, at least double quantities have to be fed to ensure an adequate intake of protein. If this is not done, the animal is continually hungry.

On the rare occasions when my own dogs (normally fed on red meat and vegetables) have to eat canned meat, they never seem satisfied.

(Cairns, Jack Russells, etc) require a daily quantity of at least one pound (0·454 kg), whereas the larger breeds (Alsatian, Labrador, etc) require a minimum of three pounds (1·36 kg). A good way of determining the correct bulk is to estimate it at approximately one twentieth of the dog's body weight.

Correct feeding gives any dog the maximum chance of being and remaining healthy, but there are two other important factors, neglect of either of which can not only damage the dog's health but also make its life a misery. They are Housing and Exercise, dealt with in the following chapter.

2
Housing and Exercise

IF, as most do, the dog lives in the house of its owner, then there is little problem though there are two important points to remember.

1. If possible avoid sleeping the dog in a cold kitchen or scullery after it has spent the entire evening luxuriating in the warm lounge; the change of temperature can and most certainly will trigger off chills, pneumonia, gastro-enteritis and fibrositis.

2. Try to have the dog's bed situated so that the air space above his sleeping back is not too high, e.g. the bottom of a cupboard is the ideal *(photo 1)*. In this way the heat from the dog's own body will provide an all-night constant temperature.

Dogs housed outside, such as farm dogs, provide a special problem.

The ideal type of kennel or housing for the outside dog is illustrated *(photo 2)*. It

1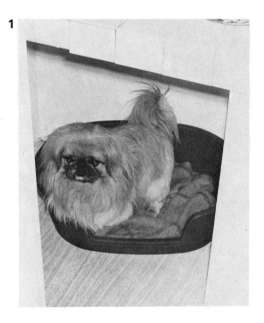

2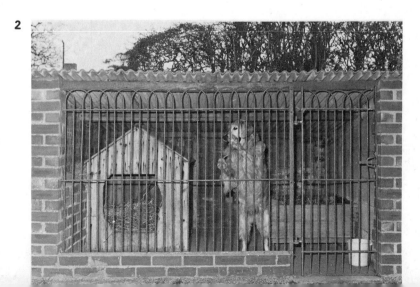

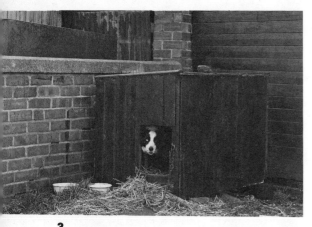

3

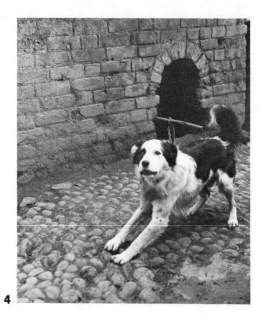

4

comprises a 'kennel within a house'. The external house faces south, there is ample exercise space within and a straw bed is provided outside the kennel so that the dog will not have to lie on the concrete. Such a building is not expensive. Another advantage is that it allows the dogs a full view of the entire farmyard. Insulation is provided by the air space between the asbestos and the roof of the kennel. The bed is insulated and covered with abundant fresh straw.

The traditional type of farmyard kennel *(photo 3)* has much to commend it. It is small, well insulated and the entrance can be sited to suit the weather. It is most

important to keep it draughtproof and this can easily be done by nailing a layer of roofing felt to the outside walls.

Another type of house which makes an ideal kennel, provided it is facing south and the floor is insulated and the roof not too high, is also illustrated *(photo 4)*.

If the dog is kept solely as a 'watch', then here *(photo 5)* is something of the ideal night quarters. During the day he should be free to roam the farm or garden at will. These night quarters comprise an extensive wired-in exercise yard and an ultra-cosy two-compartment insulated kennel made from an old fowl pen.

EXERCISE

Ample exercise is vital to health. In my opinion a dog should never be chained up. If confined for limited periods, it should be in kennels similar to those shown in photos 2 and 5.

For most pets the freedom of the garden during the day, plus a decent walk every evening and a couple of romps in the country at week-ends, provides an ideal

5

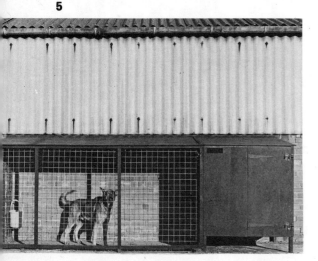

formula for health, fitness and longevity.

The freedom of the garden to my mind is vital. Far too many pets spend long days lying on the carpet or in baskets beside the fire with only ten minutes walk each night. This is not enough and inevitably leads to obesity and premature senility.

To sum up, therefore, the simple formula for maximum health in the dog is not unlike that for humans: correct feeding—warm dry sleeping quarters—and regular and adequate exercise *(photo 6)*.

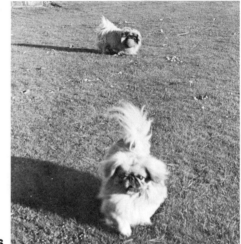

6

3
Choice of Dog

WHICH TYPE of dog is best—the pedigree animal or the mongrel?

The Pedigree

I would say without any hesitation that in Great Britain the only real advantage of the purebred dog (excluding three of the working breeds, Collies, Springer Spaniels and Labradors) is that it looks nice *(photo 1)*.

The blame for this must rest fairly and squarely on the shoulders of the breeders who for many years have bred for conformation and looks, with a complete disregard for the dangers of persistent inbreeding.

By and large the breeders have not only bred the brains and intelligence out of their respective breeds but they have established and are continually perpetuating congenital defects such as hip dysplasia, congenital cataract, luxating patellas, retinal atrophy, etc.

1

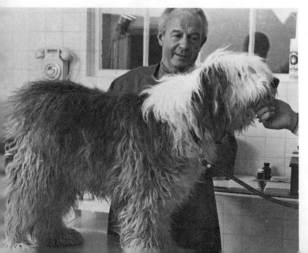

2

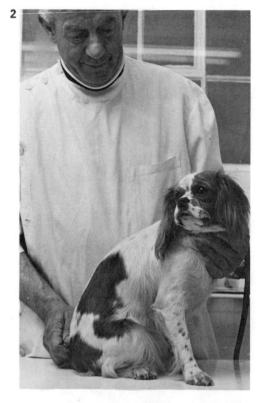

My advice, therefore, is to approach the purchase of a purebred dog with great care *(photo 2)*. If a pet only is required the less well bred the animal is, the better chance it has of being sound in body and lively and intelligent.

It is only a matter of time before some enlightened breeder will start the creation

22

of new British breeds by selective crossing of the larger and the smaller animals. In this they will merely be following the pattern already firmly established in other species, viz. horses, cattle, sheep and pigs. In other words hybrid vigour and intelligence will become the qualities most sought after, as indeed they should be.

The Crossbred

The crossbred dog has many advantages over its purebred brother *(photo 3)*. It is usually free from congenital defects, is tougher, more intelligent, much more resistant to disease and usually lives longer.

Indiscriminately-bred mongrels, however, can be ugly and stupid, so it is probably better to purchase a cross-puppy of known origin.

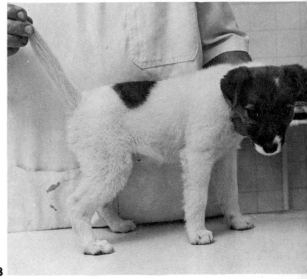

3

4
Simple Hints and First Aid

Restraint

I HAVE found that it is only rarely necessary to muzzle a dog though some veterinary surgeons do this as a routine. Few, if any, dogs are naturally vicious— they bite when spoiled, afraid or in pain and in all instances only when the handler shows hesitancy or lack of confidence. The dog's instinct, like that of other animals, tells it if an owner or veterinary surgeon is afraid of it.

However, in painful conditions some form of restraint may be advisable.

The most simple of all precautions is to put the dog on a table, preferably with a slippery surface *(photo 1)*. Several of my

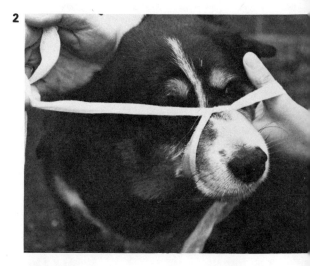

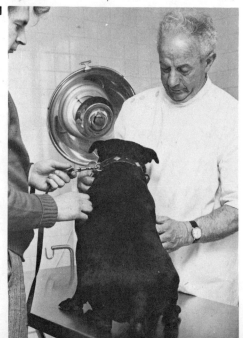

colleagues use such tables for routine examination. The uncertainty of its footing will often make the dog stand perfectly still during examination. But in any case the animal is immediately placed at a psychological disadvantage when taken off the floor.

A tape muzzle is easy to improvise and apply—all that is required is a good length of bandage, string or thin cord. A running loop is placed over both jaws with the knot at the top of the nasal region *(photo 2)*. The loop is drawn tight and the free ends of the bandage are brought round under the jaw, then crossed and brought behind the ears where they are tied tightly *(photo 3)*.

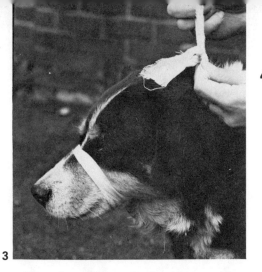

3

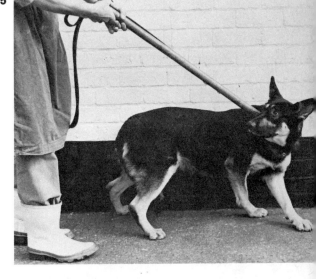

4

For the odd aggressive dog a 'dog catcher' is invaluable. This comprises a long strong but hollow metal tube through which a cord or cable is looped with the loop at one end of the tube and the free ends at the other. The loop is placed over the dog's head *(photo 4)* and tightened around the neck. This provides a rigid hold which facilitates muzzling or allows the rest of the body to be handled with reasonable safety *(photo 5)*.

In accident cases, when the dog may be painfully injured though conscious, a wise precaution is to throw a rug or coat over his head region before attempting to pick him up.

First-aid Hints

CAR ACCIDENTS

Cover the dog with a coat or rug and get it to a veterinary surgeon as quickly as possible *(photo 6)*. Leave the examination and treatment entirely to the veterinary surgeon.

5

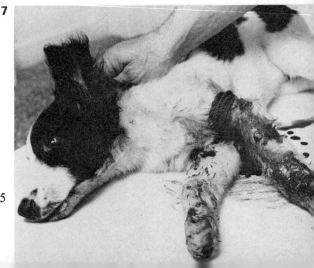

HAEMORRHAGE

If a leg is bleeding badly apply a simple tourniquet above the wound before bandaging but never leave a tourniquet on longer than 20 minutes *(photo 7)*. A

6

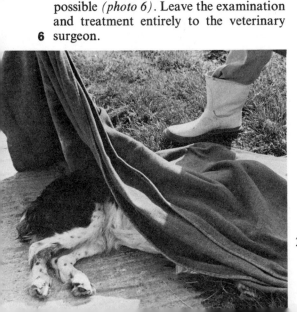

7

badly bleeding wound will always require stitching, so get the dog to a veterinary surgeon immediately after rendering first aid.

Because of the availability of sulpha drugs and antibiotics, it is not necessary for the owner to apply a local dressing.

GIVING MEDICINE

Liquid medicine presents no problem *(photo 8)*. With or without a tape muzzle in position pour the liquid in small quantities down the inside of the lips at one side of the mouth—a teaspoonful at a time is sufficient; after each lot pince the nostrils and the dog will swallow.

Tablets are much more difficult to give and are often best crushed up in food *(photo 9)*.

To ensure the swallowing of a whole tablet it is necessary to insert it over the back of the tongue—a quick poke with the point of a finger is all that is required *(photo 10)*.

Fortunately nowadays more and more treatments comprise long-acting injections which obviate the need for tablet or medicine administration.

8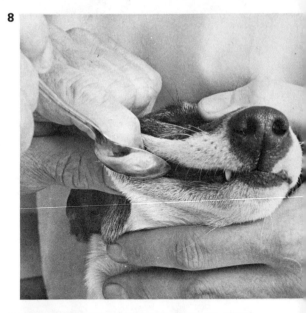

9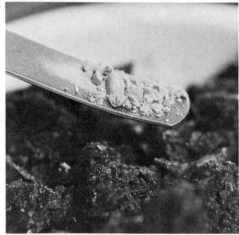

10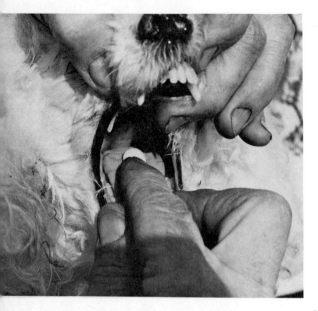

5
Preventing Disease

THERE ARE four killer diseases of dogs
and every sensible owner should protect
against these at the earliest possible
moment.

The diseases are:

1. Canine Distemper.
2. Hard Pad.
3. Virus Hepatitis.
4. Leptospiral Jaundice.

The routine drill for vaccination and
general health cover should be:

At Six Weeks of Age

Take the pup to your veterinary surgeon
(photo 1). He will examine it carefully for
fleas, lice, ear mites, and any obvious
defects such as hernias or turned-in eyelids (entropion). If any of these are present
he will put them in their true perspective,
treat the parasites, and will suggest an
appropriate time for correction of the
defects.

He will advise carefully on the feeding
(see "Feeding", page 15) and will dose for
worms, prescribing at the same time a
second dose to be given ten days later.

If there is any doubt about the puppy
being entirely confined to its own house
and garden, the veterinary surgeon will
inject a measles vaccine intramuscularly
(photo 2). This measles vaccine will give a
very good protection against distemper
and hard pad but the protection lasts only
a few weeks and the vaccine should be not
relied on as a permanent protection.

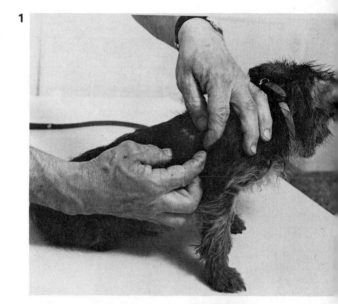

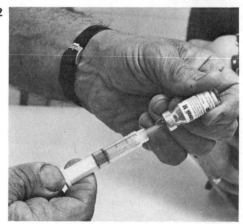

27

3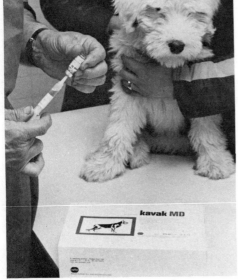

4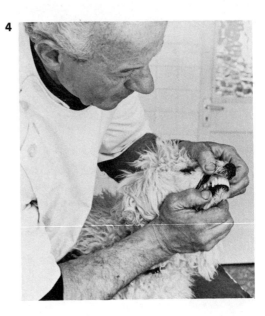

At Nine Weeks of Age

This is the correct time for the second visit to your veterinary surgeon and is probably the most important date in your puppy's life.

If the pup is completely healthy, your veterinary surgeon will inject the first dose of the comprehensive distemper and hard pad/leptospira/hepatitis vaccine *(photo 3)*. He will also instruct you to keep your pet away from other dogs until it has had the second injection.

If at nine weeks the pup is fevered or has a cough or any digestive upset, your veterinary surgeon will treat and cure the condition before inoculating.

At 11–12 Weeks of Age

Another visit to that now familiar surgery. This time the veterinary surgeon will give a booster dose against leptospirosis and will check your pup over to make sure that any of the faults found at six weeks have fully cleared.

At Six Months of Age

Another visit to the veterinary surgeon will pay handsomely. He will check the pup's mouth, making sure that the permanent teeth are replacing correctly the temporary ones, and will probably advise regular tooth scaling to avoid decay *(photo 4)*.

At the same time he will check the general condition and will prescribe the correct diet and exercise routine.

Every Year

Although some of the modern vaccines give a two-year immunity, it is best to have a booster injection against the killer diseases every 12 months.

This booster visit will give your veterinary surgeon the opportunity to check the general health of the patient and advise on teeth, ears, parasites, excess weight, etc.

To sum up, therefore, if you observe strictly this simple routine of preventive medicine your pet will be assured of a long life free from the killer diseases, any one of which would produce at the very least a long and distressing illness. In fact, despite our wide range of modern antibiotics, treatment of distemper, hard pad, hepatitis and leptospirosis is rarely successful.

6
General Knowledge

Simple Facts for Every Pet Owner and Breeder

Why do dogs eat grass (photo 1)?
This is an instinctive seeking after vitamins and minerals which are not always contained in the diet.

Why do they sometimes vomit after eating grass?
Dogs vomit easily and the sharp edges of the grass tend to produce a reflex irritation at the back of the mouth or throat.

Can bitches be artificially inseminated?
Yes—the technique is quite simple and highly successful.

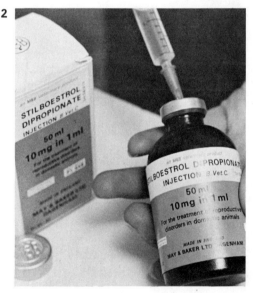

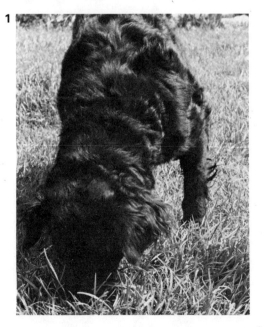

The bitch has 'stolen' the dog—can anything be done?
Yes—you have 36–48 hours in which to get the bitch to a veterinary surgeon. He will inject a large dose of female hormone (usually a drug called stilboestrol) which will prevent conception *(photo 2)*.

Do bitches abort?
Abortion in the bitch is not common but it can occur due to infection, e.g. Herpes and Virus Hepatitis. Also simple miscarriages do occur and occasionally there occurs death and reabsorption of the minute puppies.

3

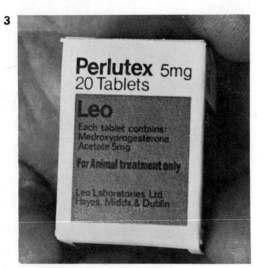

Perlutex 5mg
20 Tablets

Leo

Each tablet contains:
Medroxyprogesterone
Acetate 5mg

For Animal treatment only

Leo Laboratories Ltd.
Hayes, Middx. & Dublin

4

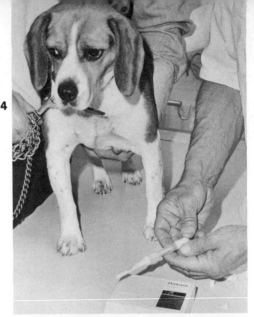

Do bitches retain their afterbirth?
Very rarely. When they do it is nearly
always only *one* afterbirth, viz. that of the
last pup born. Skilled veterinary attention
should be sought at once.

Are contraceptives available for bitches?
Certain hormone tablets can be given
daily throughout the heat period *(photo
3)*. In my experience, this will prevent
the bitch holding if she is served, though
the manufacturers say the main effect
is oestrus suppression.

A hormone injection can be given one
month before the season is due. This will
prevent the bitch coming into season and
the injections can be continued throughout
the life of the bitch *(photo 4)*.

Both of these contraceptives are now
perfectly safe and many owners prefer
their use to spaying.

Vile smelling solutions available for
painting on the bitch's genitalia are of no
use whatsoever and should never be relied
on.

*Why do bitches eat the afterbirth and
should they be allowed to do so (photo 5)?*
The afterbirth contains hormonal fluids
which help in the production of milk; the
bitch should never be prevented from this
instinctive habit.

5

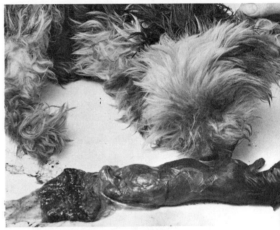

*A small lump on the pup's navel—should
anything be done about it (photo 6)?*
This is usually a small rupture (hernia). It
is a common congenital weakness often
transmitted by the dog, called an umbilical
hernia. THE VAST MAJORITY CON-
TAIN ONLY A SMALL PIECE OF FAT
OR MESENTERY AND ARE BEST
LEFT ENTIRELY ALONE.

6

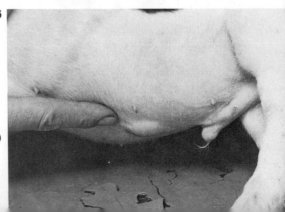

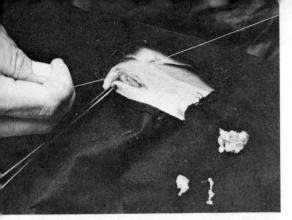

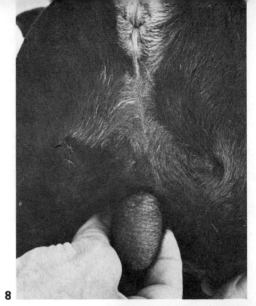

7 If the lump is large and contains intestine, the veterinary surgeon will operate when the pup is old enough *(photo 7)*.

One testicle only?
Such a dog is known as a monorchid or cryptocid *(photo 8)*. The missing testicle will be in the abdomen and should be removed surgically, if not, it may become cancerous in later life. If a breeding dog, veterinary advice should be sought. A testosterone implant may be necessary *(photo 9)*.

8

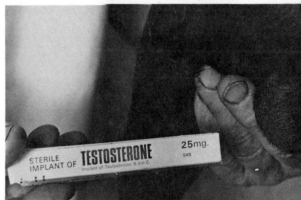

Travel sickness—can anything be done about it?
Modern tranquillisers prescribed by your veterinary surgeon will completely control this problem *(photo 10)*.

9

10

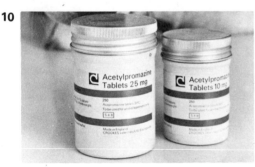

Shock! When does it occur and how is it best treated?
Shock is a state of what we call anaphylaxis. *(photo 11)*. It occurs after car or other accidents. It can also occur after certain injections if the dog is allergic to the substance used (e.g. certain anti-sera and antibiotics). It is always best treated by a

My dog shivers for no apparent reason—is there anything I should do about it?
If your dog is a Poodle that has been clipped in the winter time, then small wonder it shivers—stop the winter clipping.

However, some dogs, especially Terriers, shiver for no apparent reason. The habit should be disregarded completely unless the dog goes off its food or starts to vomit.

11

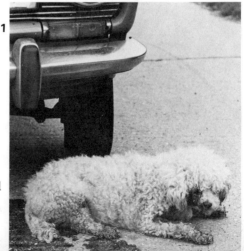

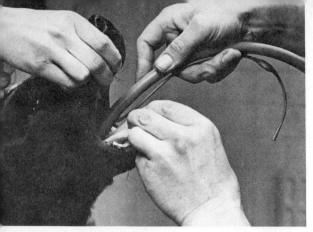

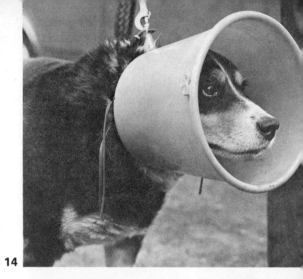

12 veterinary surgeon, who will inject a drug called an antihistamine.

14

What anaesthetics are used when operating? Is there any anaesthetic risk?
Modern veterinary practice now offers the same range of ultra-safe anaesthetics that are used in humans *(photo 12)*.

Despite this there is always a slight risk though this is absolute minimal; in my experience less than 0·001 per cent.

Can dogs be given intravenous drips and blood transfusions (photo 13)?
Yes, and they often are. Blood grouping

13

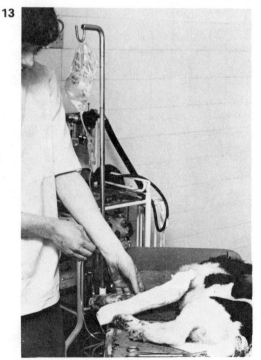

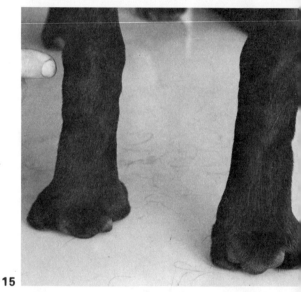

15

apparently presents little problems and 'blood banks' are available in some practices.

After operations, what is the best method of stopping the dog biting the stitches?
By far the most satisfactory idea is to fit a plastic bucket over the dog's head as illustrated *(photo 14))* It doesn't interfere with his eating or sleeping, but it stops wound biting and completely protects operation wounds around the eyes and ears. The bucket is tied to the collar.

What is kennel lameness (photo 15)?
A term used to describe lameness due to

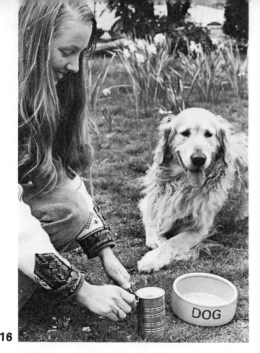

16

dietetical deficiency resulting from prolonged feeding of nothing else but dog biscuits. It can be quickly remedied by adding meat and green vegetables to the diet.

Are canned foods ever dangerous (photo 16)?
Yes! If a dog is fed *exclusively* on tinned meat for six months, a serious vitamin B_1 deficiency can develop which may produce heart failure and death.

It is always advisable therefore to subsidise and vary your dog's diet when the only source of meat is from a tin.

What causes a 'staring' coat (photo 17)?
The cause can be complex but one simple

17

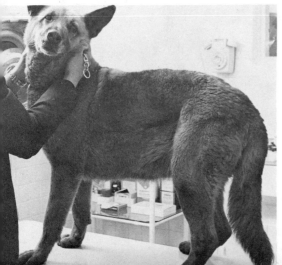

predisposing factor is a lack of fat in the diet. To offset this, feed daily a small piece of bread and butter.

Do dogs get tetanus (i.e. lockjaw)?
Very rarely: when it does occur however it is usually fatal. It is probably safest therefore to have a protective inoculation especially after road accidents.

Do dogs get 'impetigo'?
Yes. Impetigo describes an area of apparently painless pustules and is liable to occur whenever the resistance is lowered. For example, it is seen in pups during teething, especially when they are heavily infected with roundworm. It also occurs in distemper (see 'Distemper', page 84).

It is caused by a micrococcus and usually clears up on its own as soon as the dog's condition gets back to normal.

Ticks? Can a dog be infested?
The answer is no, though often one or several sheep ticks attach themselves to a dog's skin and swell up to look just like grey warts *(photo 18)*.

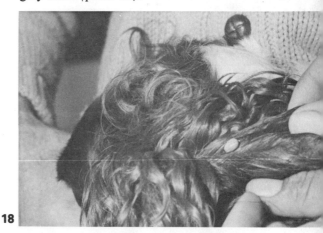

18

The veterinary surgeon will remove the ticks by anaesthetising them with ether.

Don't be tempted to pull the tick from the dog or the head portion of the parasite may be left buried in the skin and cause an abscess.

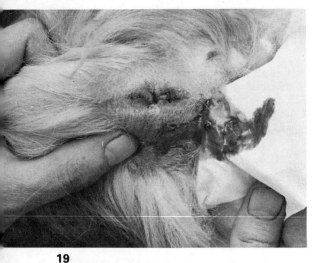

19

What is an abscess (photo 19)?
An accumulation of pus, usually under the skin, caused by bacteria gaining entry through a scratch or wound and starting to multiply. The bacteria destroy tissue and it is the dead tissue which changes into pus.

Most abscesses form in six or seven days and are ready for lancing around the tenth day. Treatment should always be left to your veterinary surgeon.

Small lumps occasionally appear at the root of the dog's hairs (photo 20)—are these abscesses?
They are probably simple sebacious cysts but your veterinary surgeon will advise you.

What is a 'honey cyst'?
A honey cyst is the name given to a cyst formed by a blockage in a salivary duct. The honey cyst or 'ranula' forms under the dog's tongue or jaw and its diagnosis and treatment must always be left to the veterinary surgeon.

Can dogs get heat stroke?
Yes—if they go to sleep in a strong sun. They stagger and behave queerly when they try to stand up; the body temperature can rise to 108°F (45°C).

The simple first-aid remedy is to throw a bucket of cold water over the animal.

When should a dog's nails be clipped?
The correct length of a dog's nail is level with the pad.

Clipping (*photo 21*) should be done only by a veterinary surgeon or experienced dog breeder because of the danger of cutting the so-called 'quick'. If the quick is ever cut during nail-clipping, the dog will never forget and will be unwilling to co-operate

21

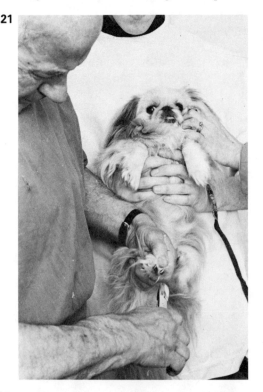

20

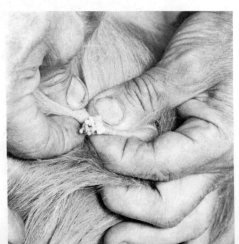

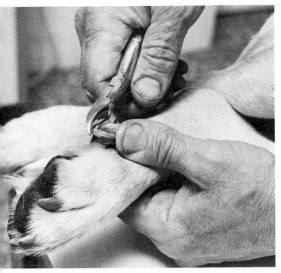

22

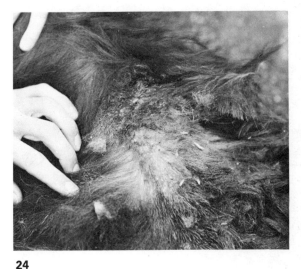

24

at future nail-cutting sessions. Dew claws have to be clipped regularly *(photo 22)*.

Dirty backsides—what causes them?
These are seen chiefly in long-coated breeds, e.g. Pekes *(photo 23)*.

In my experience they can be prevented by regular clipping of the hair around the anus and under the tail. This routine is especially important in old dogs and during the summer because of the danger of myiasis (i.e. maggots) *(photo 24)*. A dirty backside on a dog is an ideal site for the blow-flies to lay their eggs.

Euthanasia—what is the modern method?
Most veterinary surgeons will inject a tranquilliser or immobilising drug when the dog is admitted, to ensure absolutely no distress.

The euthanasia is completed by injecting intravenously a large dose of a pentobarbitone solution *(photo 25)*. Death is virtually instantaneous and absolutely painless.

25

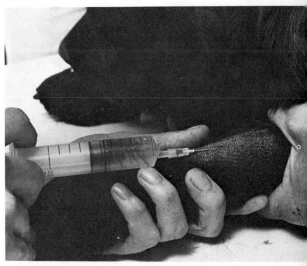

23

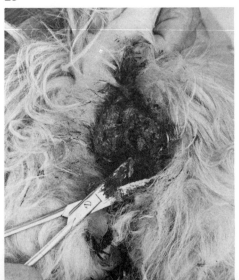

THE BITCH

7
The Bitch

Breeding

DURING HER lifetime an entire bitch (one that has not been spayed) comes in season twice a year—in the spring and in the autumn.

The season or 'heat period' lasts for approximately three weeks.

The first sign is usually the sudden appearance of one or several unwanted 'male friends' whose instinct appears almost uncanny.

The bitch's vulva swells and there is usually a bloody discharge which lasts for up to nine days *(photo 1)*.

Ovulation, i.e. the discharge of eggs from the ovaries into the fallopian tubes, occurs during the five days following, i.e. from the tenth to the fourteenth day inclusive. Obviously where breeding is practised, this is the best time to put the bitch to the dog. In fact the bitch will not take the dog until the tenth day.

Natural Service

When a bitch is ready for service she stands quietly with her tail raised.

After the first few 'thrusting' movements by the dog the two animals 'tie' together and remain apparently 'stuck' for up to half an hour or even longer. When the dog is 'thrusting' he is passing spermatozoa floating in seminal fluid; when he is 'tied' he is passing his prostatic fluid which contains necessary food to keep the sperms alive and active and which stimulates the spermatozoa and helps it on its way to the uterus and fallopian tubes.

Don't panic when the dog and bitch appear 'tied' or 'stuck'. It is a perfectly natural phenomenon and indicates that the service has been a good one.

The gestation period (i.e. the time the pups are carried) is nine weeks.

1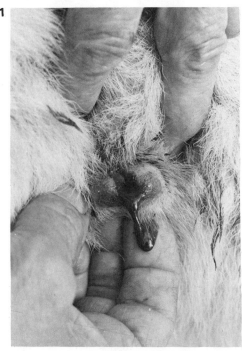

Whelping

THE BIRTH OF THE PUPS— PARTURITION *(photo 2)*

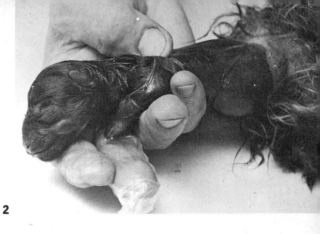

At one time it was thought that a bitch should produce her entire litter within twelve hours of the onset of labour but this time restriction is now known to be nonsense. The period required on an average from the onset of first-stage labour is from 36 to 50 hours depending on which litter is being born; obviously a first litter requires longer.

Labour in the bitch *(photo 3)*, as in humans and all other animals, is divided into three stages.

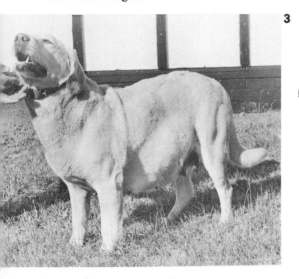

First-stage labour is when the neck of the uterus is opening up ready for the delivery of the pups. Uterine contractions occur every six or seven minutes but these are comparatively mild. They exert intermittent pressure of the uterine contents on the cervix or neck of the uterus (womb) and this, plus passive hormonal relaxation, causes the cervix to gradually open up.

This process can take up to 24 hours (as it can in humans). During this time the bitch will behave abnormally *(photo 4)* She will pace around restlessly, make beds,

growl and refuse to eat or drink (though some bitches at this time show a voracious appetite). *During this period there is absolutely nothing to worry about.*

Second-stage labour starts when the cervix is fully dilated. It comprises the actual delivery of the pups and is a much more settled and serious business. The bitch will be flat out on one side and start to strain or 'bear down' heavily. A watery or greenish discharge is usually seen at this stage, followed by the pup *(photo 5)*.

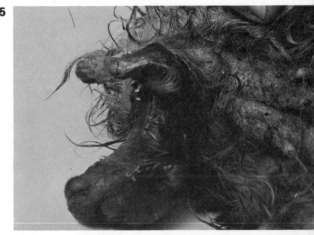

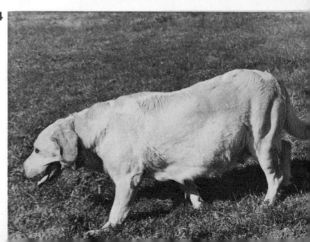

39

WHEN SECOND-STAGE LABOUR STARTS, LEAVE THE BITCH ABSOLUTELY ALONE. MOST OWNERS, ESPECIALLY WITH A FIRST LITTER, KEEP DISTURBING THE BITCH BY PEEPING OR TALKING—THIS ONLY DELAYS THE NATURAL PROCESS.

7

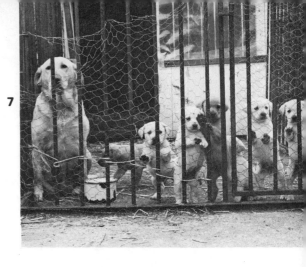

Once the bitch has started in second-stage labour leave her absolutely alone for eight hours. If after that length of time no pup has appeared, then send for your veterinary surgeon immediately but *never panic*.

Third-stage labour involves the passing of the final afterbirth *(photo 6)*. Each pup has a separate uterine attachment and set of membranes (afterbirth) and usually it is passed more or less immediately after the pup.

The answers to these queries are:

In breeding kennels the bitch should be kept in her own pen *(photo 7)* but a special insulated whelping box with a lid should be provided. It has been established beyond any doubt that one of the chief causes of puppy loss is hypothermia or loss of heat after birth—where no heating or insulation is provided this heat loss can be up to $20°F (-7°C)$.

Where the bitch is housed at home she should be allowed to whelp at least in her own environment *(photo 8)*. If an attempt is made to house her in strange surroundings the bitch will not settle, the births will be delayed and the entire litter probably lost.

An ideal spot is the bottom of a cupboard

6

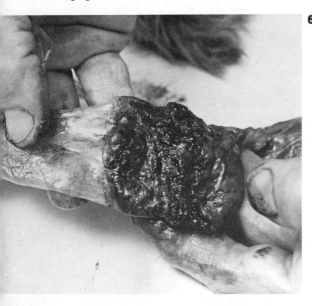

Questions I am often asked are:
Where should the bitch have her pups?
Does she require special heating?
Should the pups be taken away as they
   are born?
What should the bitch eat?
What is the best age to breed?
When is a bitch too old to breed?

8

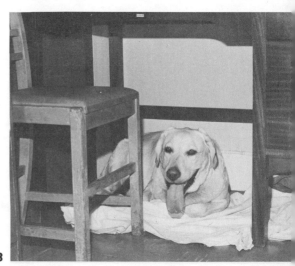

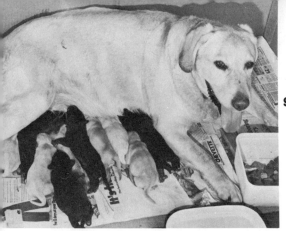

9 Whelping as in birth of humans and all classes of animals is the most natural phenomenon in the world and only rarely is help needed.

in the kitchen and a comfortable bed should be provided there from the moment the bitch has been served. Most kitchens are now heated; if this is not the case provide a box which can be covered over at night or some form of heating during the whelping and for at least a fortnight afterwards *(photo 9)*.

Interfere with the bitch as little as possible and *do not remove the pups as they are born.*

During gestation (i.e. while carrying the pups) and after parturition the bitch requires the best of protein feeding and that means as much red meat as possible, eggs, cheese, and white meat all provide valuable substitutes. The old-fashioned idea that the bitch after whelping should be fed a sloppy milk diet to make milk is absolute nonsense—protein is the vital feed in the production of milk and the ideal protein for the carnivorous dog is meat (see 'Feeding', page 15).

The best age to let the bitch have her first litter is when she is two years old. A bitch is too old to have a first litter with safety at five years.

To sum up, therefore, the advice to the inexperienced particularly is to allow the bitch to whelp in her own environment on a constantly warm bed, have ample patience, and *never interfere or sit and watch the bitch during her labour and NEVER PANIC.*

Telephone the veterinary surgeon only if no pup has appeared after several hours of intensive straining, but don't worry if he takes an hour or two to get to you.

ECLAMPSIA

After whelping, at any time during the suckling period a bitch is liable to have an attack of parturient eclampsia, particularly with a large litter.

Cause
The simple term for this condition is 'milk fever' and it is due to a deficiency of calcium. Obviously a large litter places a great strain on the mother's capacity to continue to supply calcium for the development of the puppies' bones and teeth, particularly since she has already been pouring supplies into them throughout the entire gestation period.

Symptoms
The bitch starts to act queerly—she becomes dazed, restless and stumbles about. She then goes down as though in a fit, lies on her side, trembling violently and stiffens out *(photo 10)*. She starts paddling or kicking violently.

The spasm passes off but is repeated again and again with brief intervals be-

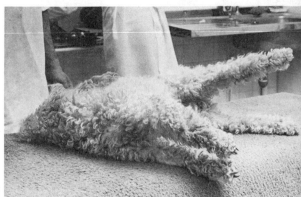

10

tween, and if not treated fairly promptly, the bitch will die from exhaustion or heart failure.

Treatment
Get the bitch to a veterinary surgeon immediately, no matter what time of the night or day. This is one condition that no veterinary surgeon will refuse to turn out of his bed for.

Injections of calcium with or without sedatives invariably produce a spectacular recovery *(photo 11)*.

Usually it is necessary, after an attack, to ration the milk supply to the pups but your veterinary surgeon will advise on this point.

Personally I advise 24 hours away from the pups followed by three days of ten-minute suckling periods every four hours before returning to full-time suckling. If the pups are old enough to lap, I start the weaning process immediately.

MASTITIS
Mastitis means inflammation of the mammary gland or glands *(photo 12)*.

Cause
It is caused by bacterial infection, the bacteria usually gaining entry through

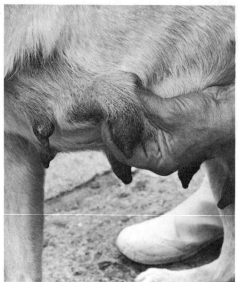

scratches or wounds in the teats. These wounds are caused by hungry pups and are most likely to occur when the bitch is short of milk (e.g. when she is not getting enough protein in her diet.)

Symptoms
The first sign is restlessness. Instead of lying contentedly suckling her pups the bitch will continually leave them. She will most likely run a fever and will probably

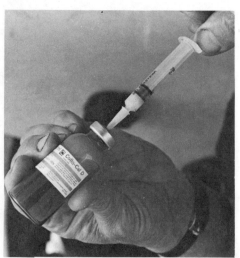

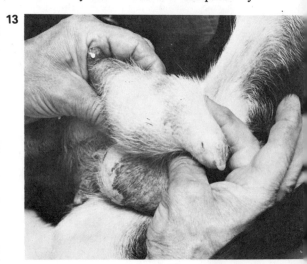

42

go off her food. Examination will show a hot painful and markedly swollen gland or glands *(photo 13)*.

Treatment
Call in your veterinary surgeon at once. If the condition is not brought under control quickly, all the milk will disappear and the entire litter may be lost.

Fortunately mastitis in the bitch responds rapidly to modern antibiotic therapy, and prompt treatment in my experience is invariably successful.

Prevention
Plenty of protein in the bitch's diet both before and after whelping.

METRITIS
Metritis simply means inflammation of the uterus and occurs after whelping.

Cause
Dead pups, retention of an afterbirth or injury during whelping.

Symptoms
There is usually a foetid discharge *(photo 14)*. The bitch will go off her food, her milk may disappear, and she will run a high temperature of around 105°F (40·5°C) or 106°F (41°C) (normal temp. 101·5°F).

Treatment
Immediate veterinary attention, otherwise the litter may be lost. The veterinary surgeon will probably swab the discharge and have the infection typed in a laboratory, but will provide an immediate powerful cover of broad spectrum antibiotics or supha drugs to control the fever *(photo 15)*. Treatment is usually successful but has to be thorough if the bitch's future breeding potential is to be protected. Also neglect at this stage can lead to pyometra (see 'Pyometra', page 48).

15

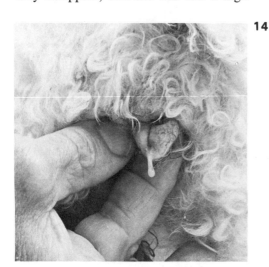

14

General Advice After Whelping
When everything is normal the bitch will stay with her pups and protect them jealously. She will eat and drink ravenously or at least normally.

Should she go off her food or become restless in any way, call your veterinary surgeon immediately. You may have an early-stage eclampsia, mastitis or metritis, and prompt treatment of any one of these will save the litter.

43

8
Caesarian Section

CAESARIAN SECTION is required only occasionally and your veterinary surgeon must always be allowed to judge when it is necessary.

Personally I have found it indicated when a pup is wrongly presented early in labour. A prompt 'caesar' provides the maximum chance of a live litter. I do not like whelping forceps; their use produces an inflammatory oedema of the vagina and slows or stops the delivery of the remaining pups.

If I cannot correct the presentation by using my fingers *(photo 1)*, and perhaps

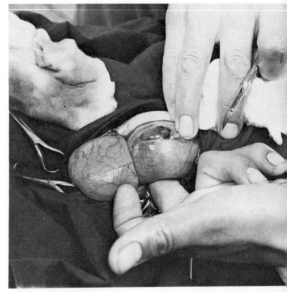

2

1

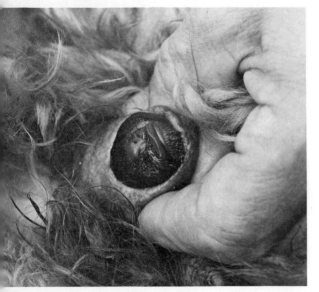

an old-fashioned button hook to bring the legs forward, then I advise a caesarian section.

The Operation

A caesarian section can be performed in mid-line or through the flank. Personally I prefer the mid-line.

The uterus is exposed and a controlled incision made in the body *(photo 2)*. Each pup is then gently manoeuvred into the body and through the opening *(photo 3)*.

To remove the afterbirth, the firm band

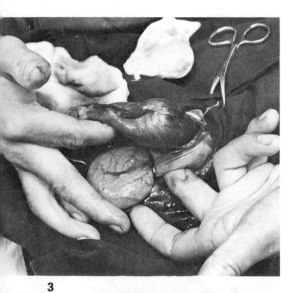

3

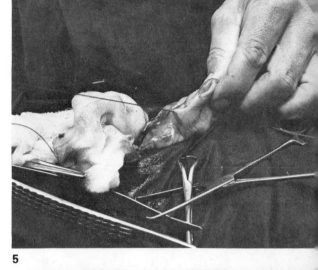

5

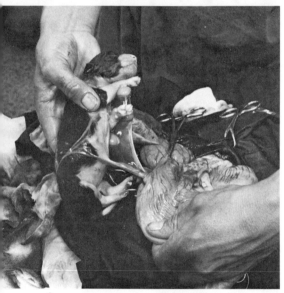

4

of the uterus where the pup has lain is squeezed tightly with the left hand then relaxed, at the same time the afterbirth is pulled gently with the right hand *(photo 4)*.

The incision is then closed by what we call a continuous Lembert suture bringing the peritoneal surfaces on each side of the wound together *(photo 5)*.

The peritoneum and abdominal muscles

are closed by a continuous catgut suture and the skin wound sealed off with nylon or special material called Dexon which does not have to be removed.

Complete healing is obtained in ten days.

Certainly at all times, caesarian section can be embarked upon with complete confidence *(photo 6)*.

45

9
False Pregnancy

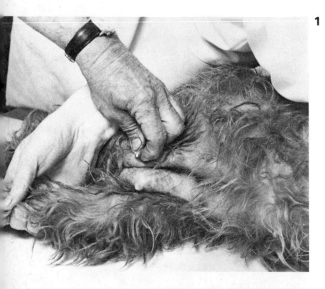

1 OCCASIONALLY A bitch will exhibit all the signs of first-stage labour, viz. making beds, carrying toys about, squealing and going off food even though she has never been to the dog. The udder fills up with milk and often the milk will drip from the teats *(photo 1)*. If not treated, the symptoms may persist for a week or ten days.

Treatment
The veterinary surgeon will inject and prescribe oral hormones *(photos 2 and 3)*.

Since false pregnancy is most common in maiden bitches, a cure may be effected by allowing the bitch to have a litter provided she is not too old. In my experience four to four and a half years is about the oldest that one might expect a bitch to have a first litter without complications, always remembering that one year of a dog's life is equal to seven years of a human.

The only infallible cure, however, for persistent false pregnancies is an ovariohysterectomy (see 'Pyometra', page 48).

2

3

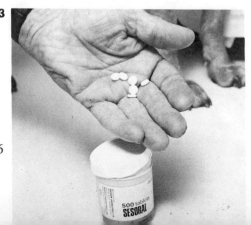

10

Cystic Ovaries

CYSTIC OVARIES are uncommon in the bitch.

Cause
Cysts form in the ovaries when the capsules (follicles) containing the eggs fail to rupture.

Symptoms
The bitch is perpetually in season.

Treatment
Removal of the ovaries by the operation of ovariotomy. This operation can be performed comfortably through the bitch's flank.

Personally I always prefer to do a complete ovario-hysterectomy, i.e. remove the entire uterus as well as the ovaries; this avoids uterine trouble later in life *(photo 1)*.

Will a Cystic Bitch Hold to the Dog?
It is extremely unlikely since the cyst or cysts interfere with the natural sexual cycle.

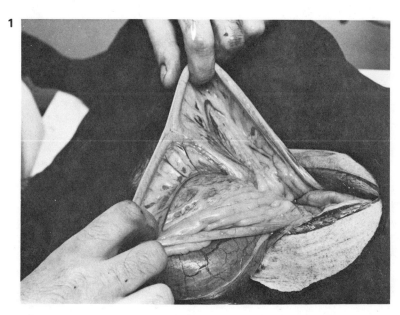

11
Pyometra

Pus in the Uterus (Womb)

PYOMETRA IS seen chiefly in maiden bitches and usually later in life (*photo 1*).

Symptoms
These often develop shortly after a season which might be described as irregular, though they can occur at any time.

There are two types—closed pyometra and open pyometra—the only difference being that a discharge, which may or may not be offensive, is seen in an open pyometra (*photo 2*).

2

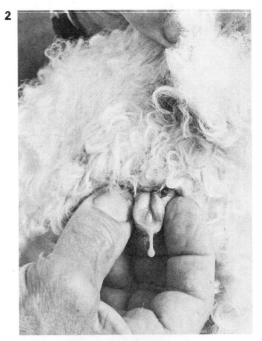

1

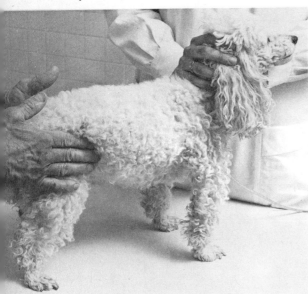

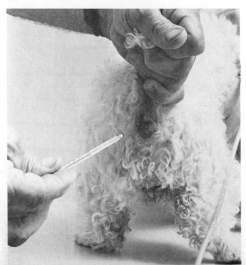

3

The first sign is that the bitch goes off colour and starts to drink excessively. She may run a high temperature but usually doesn't *(photo 3)*.

In open pyometra there is a vaginal discharge; in closed the bitch's abdomen starts to swell up markedly.

If neglected at this stage, the patient becomes toxic and starts to vomit persistently.

Treatment

The only satisfactory treatment is the operation of complete ovario-hysterectomy and the sooner it is performed the better *(photo 4)*.

Done prior to the toxic syndrome, ovario-hysterectomy in pyometra is virtually 100 per cent successful.

Where the bitch is toxic and vomiting, the success rate goes down to 50 per cent or even less.

4

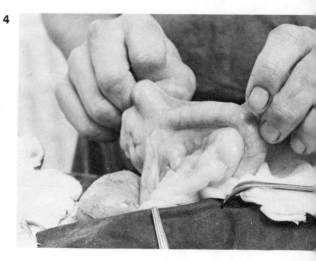

Prevention

If a bitch is being spayed, always insist on a complete ovario-hysterectomy.

If kept entire, allow at least one litter of pups.

CUSHING'S SYNDROME

This is a condition that can be mistaken for pyometra, though it occurs in the dog as well as in the bitch.

Cause

A tumour in the adrenal gland or an excess growth of the adrenal glands due to a malfunction of the pituitary gland at the base of the brain.

Symptoms

Excessive drinking and urination. The abdomen may swell up and in the bitch the heat periods may be abnormal. There is a thinning of the coat or patches of baldness *(photo 1)*.

Treatment

The diagnosis and treatment of this condition is very much a job for the veterinary surgeon.

1

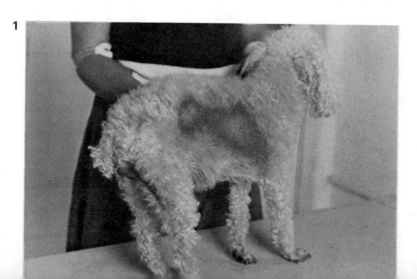

12

Uterine Polypi and Other Disorders

VERY OCCASIONALLY polypi—wart-like growths on long stalks—form in the uterus. The cause is unknown.

Symptoms
Hard lumps can be palpated in the uterus. There may be a bloody discharge but the bitch is otherwise completely normal.

Treatment
Complete ovario-hysterectomy.

VAGINAL TUMOURS AND WARTS
Occasionally one or other of these may protrude from the vulva usually of an old bitch *(photo 1)*.

Treatment comprises surgical removal by thermocautery, done of course only by a veterinary surgeon.

CANCER OF THE BITCH'S GENITAL TRACT
It is my experience that, in the Midlands of England at least, while cancer is comparatively rare in the bitch genital tract, it occurs frequently in the mammary glands of bitches.

MAMMARY TUMOURS
Without doubt mammary tumours are one of the commonest conditions that we have to deal with, especially in older bitches *(photo 2)*.

1

2

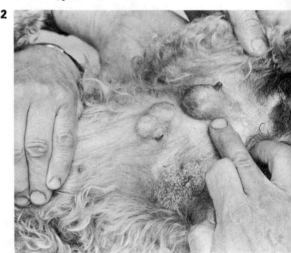

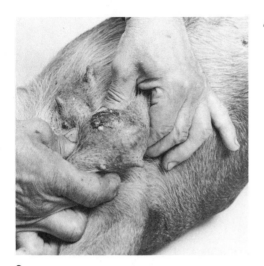

3

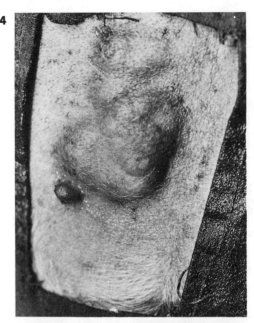

4

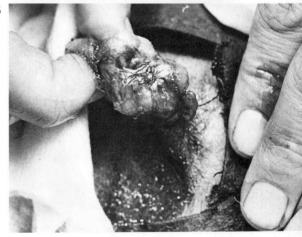

5

There are two distinct types and both are usually malignant.

The less dangerous are the circumscribed type which can be isolated with the fingers from the surrounding tissues *(photo 3)*.

The more dangerous are the diffuse type which cannot be isolated and appear to diffuse or spread into the nearby skin and muscles *(photo 4)*.

Treatment

Mammary tumours, even the small circumscribed type, should always be removed surgically as soon as they are detected. Here we veterinary surgeons follow the example of the human surgeons. The longer the tumour is allowed to remain, the greater the danger of secondary growths appearing not only in the udder but also in the lymphatic glands within the abdomen.

Hormone therapy may be tried but I have found that this predisposes to kidney trouble.

The Operation

Caught early most mammary tumours can be dissected out successfully *(photo 5)*.

Many surgeons favour the thermo-cautery for this operation. Certainly there is less danger of haemorrhage with this instrument.

Do Mammary Tumours Recur?

Some do but they can be removed a second and even a third time to allow the bitch to die of natural causes.

13
Vaginal Ailments

THE VAGINA is the muscular passage leading from the cervix to the vulva. In the bitch it is approximately two to three inches long. Disorders that affect the vagina (and the vulva) are:

VAGINITIS
Vaginitis simply means inflammation of the lining of the vagina.

Cause
Specific cause is a bacterium, but the predisposing cause is usually an injury caused by a dog's penis or by a difficult whelping.

Symptoms
The bitch shows considerable discomfort and may repeatedly try to strain as though

1

in labour. There may be a red or yellow discharge. An examination using a vaginal speculum (very much a job for the veterinary surgeon) shows the lining to be markedly inflamed *(photo 1)*.

Treatment
Where vaginitis is suspected, a veterinary surgeon should be consulted immediately. He will probably prescribe a course of antibiotics together with daily insertion of a pessary.

PROLAPSE
This term describes the condition where the cervix and vagina fold back on themselves and protrude from the vulva *(photo 2)*. Sometimes the bladder is included in

2

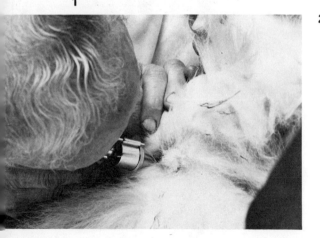

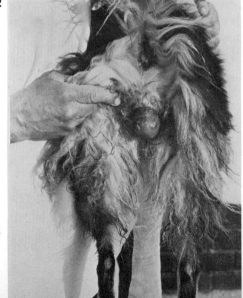

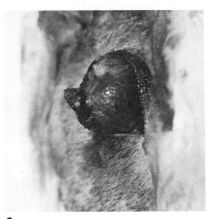

3

the prolapse and very occasionally the uterus as well.

Symptoms
A red and inflamed mass protruding from the vulva which the bitch licks incessantly *(photo 3)*.

Treatment
An immediate visit to the veterinary surgeon. He will replace the prolapse under a general anaesthetic and will suture it back in position *(photo 4)*.

4

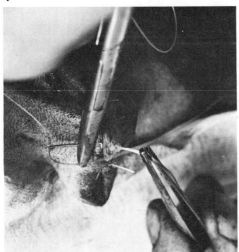

5

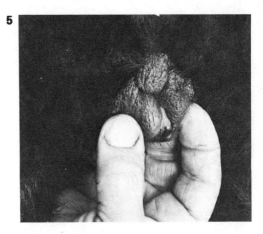

VULVITIS

This means inflammation of the vulva— the external opening into the vagina—and is usually caused during coitus or by direct injury *(photo 5)*.

It is treated with antibiotics combined with the local application of an anti-inflammatory cream.

WARTS ON THE VULVA

When warts occur at or near the vulva they are best removed since they tend to produce an irritation and incontinence *(photo 6)*. (See Warts, page 76).

6

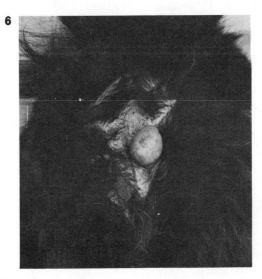

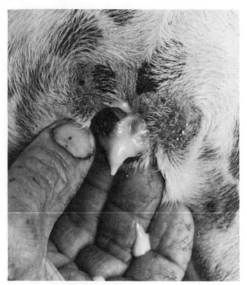

7

LEUCORRHOEA

Leucorrhoea occurs where there is a chronic vaginitis.

Symptoms

A white or yellow pus discharge persisting over a comparatively long period of time *(photo 7)*.

8

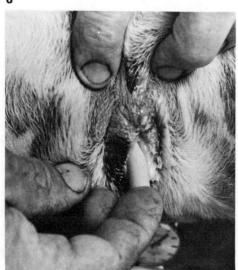

Cause

Leucorrhoea is usually secondary to an acute vaginitis and is complicated by the growth of secondary bacteria or fungi.

Treatment

This condition is often extremely difficult to clear up and treatment should only be attempted under the guidance of a veterinary surgeon, who will probably prescribe a combination of repeated irrigation, the administration of a soft tissue antibiotic or pessaries *(photo 8)*.

VENEREAL DISEASE

Fortunately venereal disease in the dog is virtually unknown. Occasionally in the spring and autumn a dog may develop a pus discharge from the sheath. This often gives rise to considerable concern by the owner but is due to a simple inflammation of the sheath (prepuce), and the bacterium concerned is usually a streptococcus which does not cause any transmissible disease.

A canine transmissible venereal tumour has been recorded but this is rare.

The discharge from the dog's prepuce *(photo 9)* often flares up secondary to sexual excitement caused by the proximity of bitches in season and it can be caused by masturbation.

Treatment

The condition rapidly clears up with local antibiotic treatment which will be prescribed by a veterinary surgeon.

9

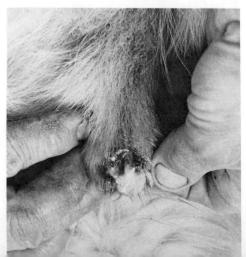

14
Spaying

SPAYING MEANS simply removing the ovaries from a bitch's abdomen so that she cannot breed. The ovaries can be taken out through the flank or along the abdominal midline. The latter site is preferable if the entire uterus is to be removed with the ovaries *(photo 1)*.

There is a great deal to be said for and against spaying. On the one hand, the operation removes the embarrassment and trouble associated with heat periods and unwanted litters which often lead to an increase in the stray dog population.

On the other hand, spaying tends to make a bitch fat and lazy.

Personally I don't like spaying. I'd prefer to see the stray dog population controlled by sterilising the males. However, if spaying has to be done, then I recommend and practise the removal of the entire uterus as well as the ovaries (see 'Ovariohysterectomy', page 49). This avoids uterine trouble later in life (see 'Pyometra', page 48).

The Best Age for Spaying

This is debatable. Many veterinary surgeons insist on the bitch having at least one heat period. I have found the best age to

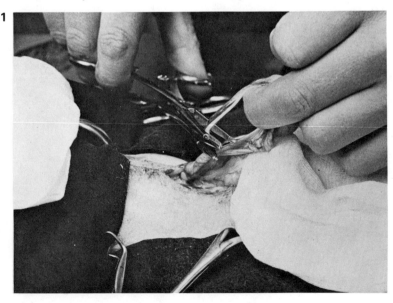

1

be six months regardless of whether the bitch has had a season or not *(photo 2)*. At six months the pup is big enough to withstand a general anaesthetic and young enough to heal rapidly and recover quickly.

Can Older Bitches by Spayed?
Certainly. The operation can be done at any time.

Some spayed bitches appear to come into season. When this happens it is due to aberrant ovarian tissue floating around in the abdomen. This is inaccessible but not dangerous since the spayed bitch will not hold to the dog.

Is Spaying Expensive?
Comparatively because it involves an abdominal operation and a general anaesthetic is required.

2

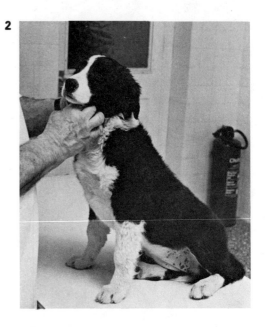

THE DOG

15
The Dog's Genital Tract

THE TESTICLES, which are contained in a sac called the scrotum, manufacture spermatozoa which are stored in the vesicula seminalis and ejaculated during coitus. The prostate gland secretes a nourishing fluid which mixes with the sperms to keep them alive.

Diseases
Prostatitis is dealt with under bowel obstruction (see page 152).

ORCHITIS
This means simply inflammation of the testicles *(photo 1)*.

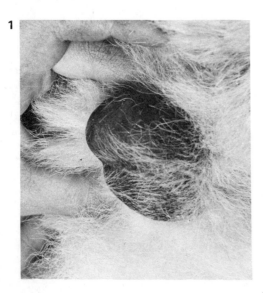

1

Cause
Usually some injury—a kick or a bruise caused during fence jumping. Very occasionally they may be infected by bacteria.

Symptoms
The testicles are usually hot and painful and the dog resents strongly their handling and examination.

If an abscess is present the dog's temperature is usually elevated to around 105°F (40·5°C).

Treatment
As a first-aid measure the testicles may be fomented with warm water containing Epsom salts (one tablespoonful to the gallon) but invariably it is best to have the condition treated by a veterinary surgeon.

He will probably inject long-acting cortisone with long-acting antibiotic and prescribe oral pain-killers or anti-inflammatory agents.

TUMOURS OF THE TESTICLE
These are not uncommon though as a rule only one testicle is involved *(photo 2)*.

Symptoms
The testicle is hard and solid and non-painful.

Treatment
Immediate surgical removal for the same reasons as described under the removal of mammary tumours.

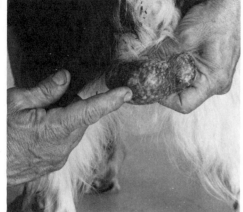

4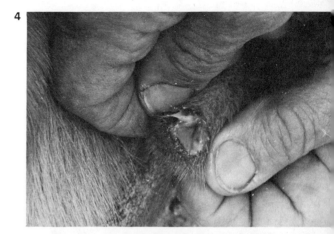

BALANITIS

This means inflammation of the end of the penis which is covered by the prepuce or sheath *(photo 3)*.

Cause

Injury, though occasionally the inside of the sheath becomes infected by bacteria.

Symptoms

In cases of injury the sheath is markedly swollen and painful.

Where infection is present the only sign may be a purulent discharge *(photo 4)*.

Treatment

The veterinary surgeon will diagnose the

5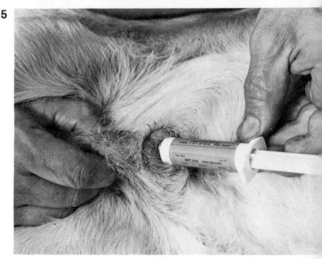

3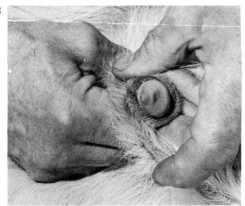

condition and prescribe the correct treatment.

Where there is a discharge he will probably take a swab and have the bacteria typed in a laboratory. He will then syringe out the sheath with the appropriate antibiotic and repeat the treatment weekly until the condition clears up *(photo 5)*.

FRACTURE OF THE OS PENIS

The dog is the only animal with a bone in

the penis, and this bone is called the *Os penis (photo 6)*.

Occasionally, and fortunately only occasionally, this bone is fractured. Personally I have seen this only twice in thirty-four years of practice.

Cause
Direct injury sustained during attempted coitus, although it may occur during a road accident or when the dog is jumping over a fence.

Symptoms
A severe swelling and acute pain. Crepitation can be detected and the diagnosis can be confirmed by X-ray.

Treatment
Very much a matter for your veterinary surgeon.

THE BULBOUS URETHRA
The penis of the dog, during erection and especially during intercourse, shows a hard round prominent swelling around the base of the *Os penis*. This is called the bulbous urethra and plays an important part in holding the dog and bitch together during intercourse *(see sketch)*.

When a dog and a bitch get locked together during coitus, it is due to a spasm of the bitch's vaginal muscle contracted around the bulbous urethra.

When they do get stuck, the best treatment is to leave the animals severely alone, for at least a few minutes. Interference by humans increases the bitch's tension and reduces the chance of relaxation of the muscle spasm. In fact the 'locking' period is natural and vital to successful mating (see 'Natural Service', page 38). However, if unduly prolonged, squat down and steady the bitch by holding her head or body until the dog disengages.

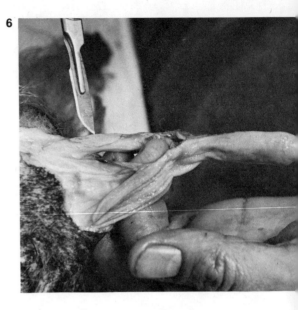

6

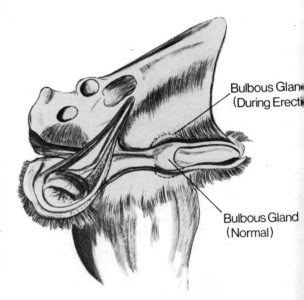

Bulbous Gland
(During Erection)

Bulbous Gland
(Normal)

16
Castration and Vasectomy

CASTRATION
CASTRATION OF the male dog involves the surgical removal of both testicles under a general anaesthetic *(photo 1)*. Both testicles are taken out through a single mid-line incision towards the base of the penis. The operation is comparatively simple and completely successful though, as with spaying, the castrated dog often tends to put on weight.

Advantages
Castration not only sterilises the dog but it stops him wandering away from home and makes him much more docile.

Disadvantage
The only disadvantage is the tendency to put on weight.

Age for Castration
Any age after six months. I have castrated a ten-year-old dog without apparent ill effect.

Vasectomy

This sterilising operation comprises the cutting of both spermatic cords in the male dog *(photo 2)*. Performed under a general or local anaesthetic it sterilises the dog without producing obesity. However, it doesn't stop the dog from wandering nor does it alter his temperament in any way.

I am convinced that compulsory mass vasectomy is the only sensible answer to the stray dog problem. Stud dogs would remain entire but under special licence only.

There can be little doubt that vasectomy is a much more satisfactory way of controlling indiscriminate breeding than spaying or castration.

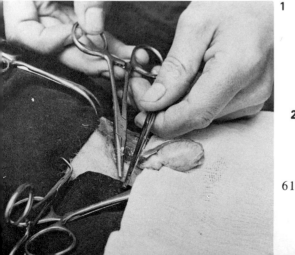

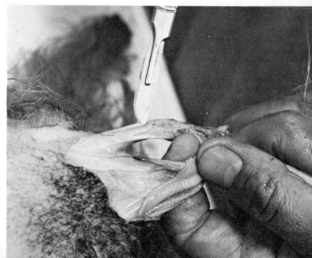

SKIN DISEASES

17
Eczema

ECZEMA IS a general term to describe inflammation of the skin.

There are five common types recognised:

Acute moist, dry, allergic (including urticaria), digital, and scrotal.

ACUTE MOIST ECZEMA

Cause

Excess feeding of carbohydrates. It is my experience that you can take any dog and by feeding exclusively high carbohydrate foods such as bread, potatoes or porridge, you can produce a moist eczema on the skin surface within a month *(photo 1)*. A

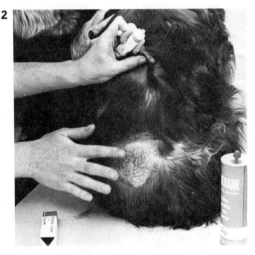

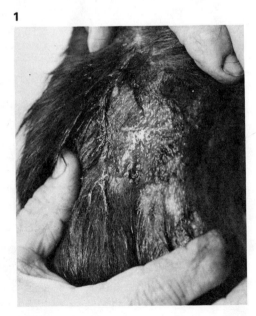

heavy infestation of fleas or lice can also produce a raw eczematous patch. Acute moist eczema can also result from a meal allergy.

Symptoms

Violent biting and scratching of a localised area. Examination reveals an acutely painful circular moist patch often infected and scabbed over *(photo 2)*. A search of the area may reveal fleas or lice as it did in this case.

Treatment

Correct the diet immediately. The veterinary surgeon will clean up and dress the lesion and will inject or provide oral antiflammatory drugs—usually cortisone. An immediate response is obtained but

IF THE DIET IS NOT CORRECTED the condition will recur.

Since the feeding of larger dogs particularly presents an economic problem, I usually advise a 50 per cent reduction in the intake of carbohydrate and an increase in the protein ration.

Moist eczematous patches can of course be caused by the persistent licking or biting of an area infected with parasites or it can occur behind the ear due to constant scratching of that area, but the veterinary surgeon will quickly spot either of these conditions and will treat them accordingly.

DRY ECZEMA

One of the most difficult skin conditions to diagnose and treat (*photo 3*).

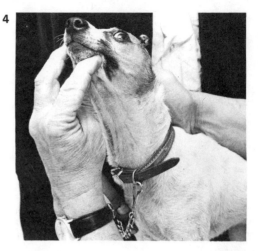

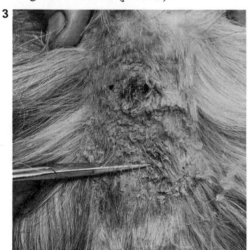

may not show a hyperaemia (a reddening of the skin surface).

Treatment

A careful examination by your veterinary surgeon (which will include skin scrapings) will be required to eliminate the other possible causes of persistent scratching (mange, fleas and lice).

Having done this, he will probably correct the diet if necessary and prescribe a course of anti-inflammatory steroids (*photo 5*).

Unfortunately treatment may have to be repeated every few months.

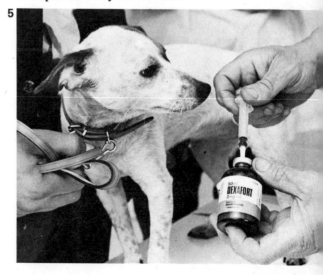

Cause

The cause is often obscure. It seems to be most common in pedigree dogs and often I think there must be a hereditary predisposition.

High starch in the diet is another contributory factor, though I often see dry eczema in dogs fed exemplarily.

Symptoms

Persistent scratching producing dry scaly areas of baldness (*photo 4*).

Close examination of the skin may or

E

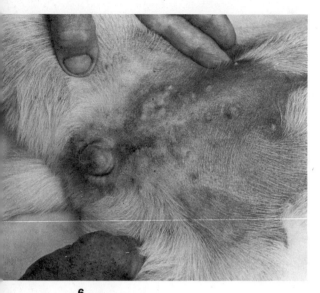

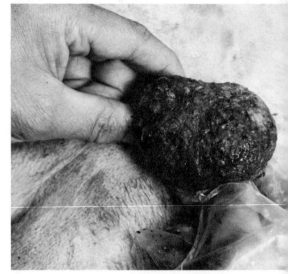

6

ALLERGIC ECZEMA

This is much more severe than simple dry eczema.

Cause

An allergy which is often impossible to pin point. In my experience the worst types are plant allergies repeatedly flaring up every time the pet roams the garden. Similar, though less severe, skin irritations can be produced by straw, wool or nylon.

Symptoms

More or less sudden appearance of an acute red rash *(photo 6)*. In the plant type the rash can extend over the entire lower part of the body with or without angry pimples, pustules or larger infected areas.

The dog scratches the rash feverishly and continuously.

Treatment

Change the dog's bedding immediately. A fresh bed of newspapers each night is ideal. Alter the route of his nightly walk and keep him out of the garden. Administer anti-inflammatory drugs such as cortisone and antihistamine under the supervision of your veterinary surgeon.

7

If you are lucky enough to identify the object, plant or material that is producing the allergy, the eczema will disappear for good. If not you will repeatedly have to treat it.

SCROTAL ECZEMA

This is a moist eczema affecting the scrotum i.e. the sack which contains the testicles *(photo 7)*.

The cause and treatment are identical to those described for acute moist eczema.

DIGITAL ECZEMA

Again, a moist eczema, this time affecting

8

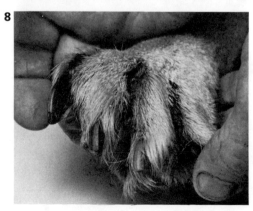

between the pads of the feet *(photo 8)*. Digital eczema is also usually due to too much carbohydrate in the diet but it may be triggered off by harvest mites (see 'Harvest Mites', page 81).

Treatment
Several cases may require kaolin poulticing but the condition usually responds rapidly to a dietetical change combined with an injection of long-acting cortisone.

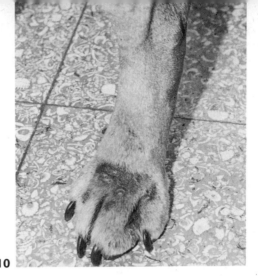

10

STAPHYLOCCAL INFECTION OF FEET

Sometimes the digits become infected and the germ most often involved is a staphylococcus.

Symptoms
Abscesses and pustules develop between the pads *(photo 9)*.

These often extend to the top surface of the foot *(photo 10)*. The patient licks the discharge and often becomes sick and unthrifty.

Treatment
The diagnosis and treatment of this condition should always be left to the veterinary surgeon.

URTICARIA OR 'BLANE'
(Nettle Rash)

One very common allergic condition which affects pups and dogs of all ages (in common with man and other animals) is the condition of urticaria or 'blane'.

Cause
Nettle rash, wasp or bee stings, fly bites and several other obscure agents. It can also be caused by indigestion.

Symptoms
The head and eyes *(photo 11)* and sometimes the neck regions swell up suddenly and alarmingly with the surface of the skin often covered in lumps. In severe cases the dog may have difficulty in breathing.

Treatment
Never panic with urticaria. If you phone or rush your pet to the veterinary surgeon, the swelling will probably have practically disappeared by the time you see him. He of course will inject antihistamine or cortisone.

I have found a useful first-aid treatment to be a pinch of baking soda (bicarbonate of soda) in a tablespoonful of cold water given by an eye dropper or teaspoon down the side of the dog's mouth.

Fortunately it appears that an attack of blane provides a degree of immunity because the condition seldom recurs.

11

9

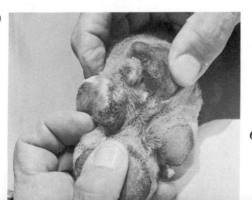

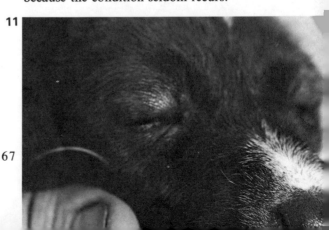

18
Mange

THERE ARE three types:
1. Sarcoptic ('Scabies').
2. Demodectic.
3. Otodectic.

The first and third are easily cleared up but the second is difficult and sometimes impossible to deal with.

SARCOPTIC MANGE

Cause

A mange mite called the *Sarcoptes scabei var canis*. This mite burrows into the surface layer of the skin and lays eggs which keep hatching out.

Symptoms

Persistent scratching with roughened bare patches appearing at the elbows *(photo 1)*, stifles and around the ears and eyes

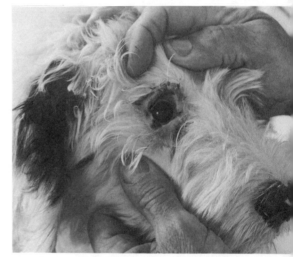

2

(photo 2). If neglected the lesions spread over the entire body. The pup or dog loses condition rapidly because it has difficulty in resting or sleeping.

The veterinary surgeon will take skin scrapings and identify the mange mite under the microscope.

Treatment

Two or three thorough skin baths containing Gammexane at intervals of seven days will invariably clear up sarcoptic mange completely.

Isolate the patient from other dogs as soon as the mange is diagnosed because it is a highly contagious condition. Wash

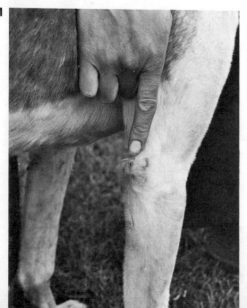

1

your hands and arms thoroughly after handling the patient, but don't panic, it only rarely affects humans.

DEMODECTIC MANGE (FOLLICULAR MANGE)

A much more serious type than sarcoptic partly because the causal parasite buries itself more deeply in the skin, but chiefly because it takes in with it a powerful bacteria called a staphylococcus. It is the staphylococcus which produces the characteristic lesions.

Cause

The *Demodex canis (see diagram)*.

Symptoms

The demodex lesions usually appear slowly with little or no itching. I've seen them most often starting in young dogs about a year old; bare patches appear round the eyes and nose or the legs and feet *(photo 3)*. These patches emit a peculiar characteristic smell.

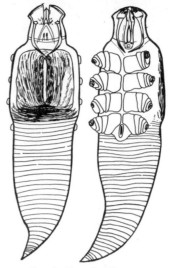

Demodex Mange Parasites
(Magnified 300 Times)

spread and the dog becomes toxic and emaciated.

The diagnosis is confirmed by the examination of skin scrapings *(photo 5)*; the demodex, more or less identical to that illustrated, can be clearly seen.

4

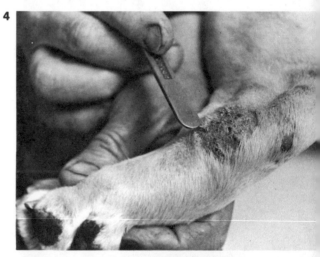

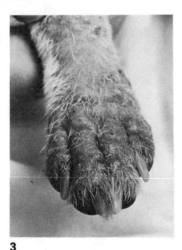

3

The surface of the lesion is usually tufted and reddened with pustules at the base of the tufts *(photo 4)*. Sometimes the skin is merely thickened and flaking but in both instances there is the typical odour.

Often, despite treatment, the patches

5

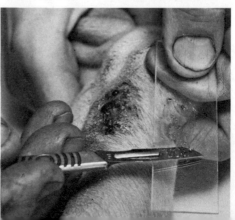

69

Treatment

Treatment is difficult, protracted and nearly always unsatisfactory because, apart from the infection, the parasite lives in a well-protected position and is difficult to reach.

When I attempt treatment I advise firstly the close clipping of the entire coat; secondly, a combined benzene hexachloride and sulphur bath; and subsequently, daily dressing of a quarter of the affected area in rotation with a powerful vile-smelling drug called Hexon 20.

If or when the disease becomes widespread, then euthanasia is indicated.

OTODECTIC MANGE
(See 'The Ear')

Cause

A mange mite called the *Otodex canis*. This mite, picked up from other dogs lives in the ear and lays its eggs in a burrow in the mucous membrane.

Symptoms

Identical to those described under 'Canker'.

Scratching and flapping the ears and shaking the head.

Diagnosis is confirmed by finding the

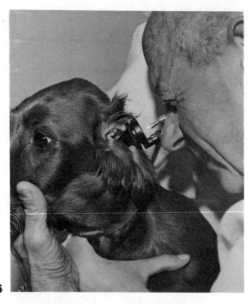

6

mite with the auroscope *(photo 6)* or in a swab examined under the low power of the microscope.

Treatment

A fourteen-day course of ear drops containing benzene hexachloride prescribed after thoroughly cleaning the ears. The ear cleaning should be done only by a veterinary surgeon since the mucous lining of the ear is delicate and easily injured.

19
Ringworm

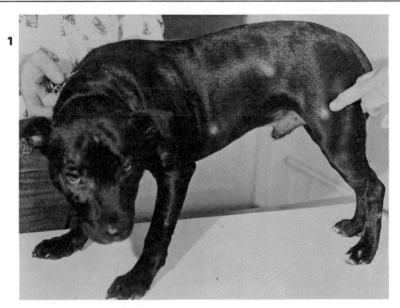

THIS COMPLAINT is fairly common in the dog *(photo 1)*.

Cause
Fungi which live either on the surface of the skin or more often in the hairs of the affected areas. There are four different types of fungi recognised in dog ringworm.

Predisposing causes are bad feeding and overcrowding (as in less reputable boarding kennels). The fungi are rapidly spread from one dog to another.

Symptoms
The first sign is scratching or biting at the skin.

Examination shows a rounded patch of crusty skin with the hairs falling out *(photo 2)*. If you scrape the lesion, the surface flakes off in scales or scabs.

Sometimes the skin is thickened, the

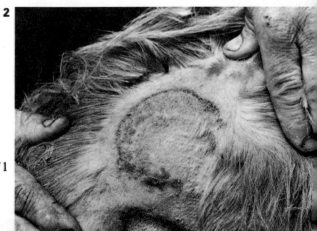

crust is yellow and its surface appears 'pitted', i.e. it has minute depressions in it.

Diagnosis should be left to your veterinary surgeon.

3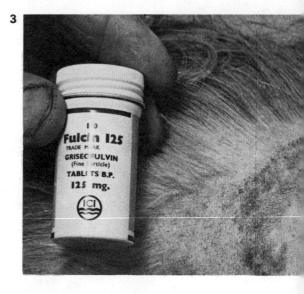

Treatment
If you have several dogs, isolate the patient immediately and during treatment don't allow the children to handle the dog, since all forms of dog ringworm can be contracted by humans.

Modern treatment is highly efficient and comprises a 7–14 day course of a drug called Griseofulvin given by the mouth *(photo 3)*.

The dog's bedding should be burned and his basket scrubbed with hot water and soda at least twice at weekly intervals.

20
Alopecia *(Loss of Hair)*

THE TERM alopecia simply means baldness *(photo 1)*.

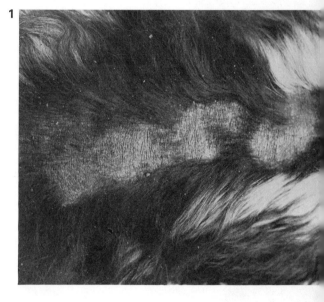

Symptoms
Loss of hair. If accompanied by itching, it is probably due to mange, eczema, ringworm or external parasites (see 'Fleas and Lice' page 78). Your veterinary surgeon will soon spot these troubles.

Several other types of baldness in the dog occur, most of which can be treated.

BALDNESS IN PUPS AT BIRTH
Cause
Often thyroid deficiency owing to lack of iodine in the food of the bitch.

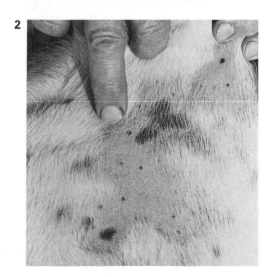

Treatment
A course of thyroid extract tablets combined with minute daily dosage of iodine often effects a cure.

BALDNESS IN OLD DOGS
Symptoms
The dog is a male and usually past middle age. The hair falls out along the back and sides *(photo 2)*. Other dogs may fuss over it as though it were a bitch and the skin becomes soft.

If neglected or undiagnosed, practically all the coat will drop out.

Cause
This is a hormonal upset.

Treatment
Castration. A complete new coat will grow within three or four months.

THYROID BALDNESS
This is seen mostly in the bitch.

Cause
Failure of the thyroid to produce sufficient quantities of thyroxine (see 'Thyroid Gland', page 131).

Symptoms
The bitch becomes dull and lacks energy. The coat becomes harsh and bare patches appear under the throat, on the flanks and behind the thighs.

Treatment
Such cases respond extremely well to daily tablets containing thyroid extract. In addition minute doses of oral iodine are indicated, though the iodine may be discontinued after a month.

HORMONAL BALDNESS IN BITCHES
This is seen after whelping.

Cause
Hormone deficiency.

Symptoms
The coat falls out in large patches, especially around the rear end and tail *(photo 3)*. There is no itching.

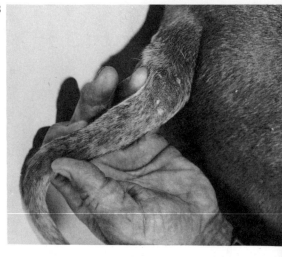

3

Treatment
Forget it and concentrate on good nutrition. The coat will grow again.

Hormone injections may be used but they sometimes upset the ovaries and jeapordise future breeding potential.

CANCER OF THE SKIN
This is uncommon but I have seen it several times in older dogs.

Symptoms
It often starts like ringworm but fails to respond to any treatment, merely spreading progressively.

Treatment
If diagnosed early, X-ray therapy may be attempted. Otherwise euthanasia is indicated.

21
Interdigital Cyst

IN MOST cases the so-called 'cyst' is in reality a small abscess *(photo 1)*. It develops between the digits of the paws.

1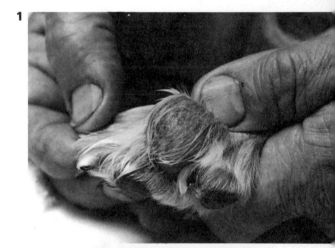

Cause

Usually an infection of the hair follicles situated between the toes, the infection gaining entrance through a scratch or cut caused by grass, sand or grit. The germs involved are chiefly the common ones, viz. streptococci and staphylococci.

Occasionally the swelling is a simple non-infected cyst.

Symptoms

The first sign is licking at the pad. Later the dog will go lame and examination of the paw will show a hard painful swelling between the digits. This comes to a head in a day or two and bursts; the dog goes sound and licks the area till it heals.

2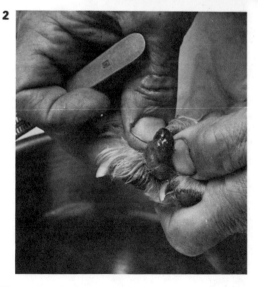

Unfortunately it is not long before another cyst appears. The dog can have a succession of them between different digits until eventually it appears to acquire a fair immunity against them.

Treatment

Hot fomentations or kaolin poultices help to bring the cyst to a head but it is always best to consult a veterinary surgeon. He will probably lance the cyst and cauterise its lining to prevent recurrence *(photo 2)*.

22
Warts

WARTS IN dogs are extremely common and may grow in clusters or singly in any part of the body *(photo 1)*.

Cause
Specific cause is unknown but warts are probably caused by a virus.

Treatment
Since warts on the dog grow very slowly (apart from mouth warts—see 'Mouth, disorders of', page 118) they rarely cause any trouble and mostly they are best left alone.

If individual warts bleed, ulcerate or become a nuisance to the dog, then they can easily be removed surgically under local anaesthesia.

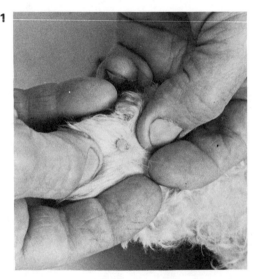

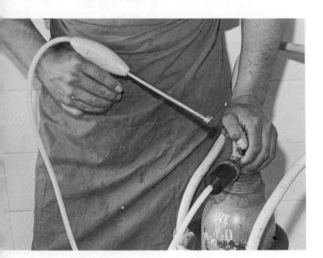

Recently I have found that probably the most effective treatment of all is cryo surgery (see anal adenoma, page 156).

The warts are frozen for varying periods, according to their size, by the special cryo surgery apparatus *(photo 2)*; the cylinder provides nitrous oxide under pressure and this reduces the temperature of the instrument to well below freezing point. The warts die and disappear. A second application is rarely necessary.

PARASITIC DISEASES

23

Parasitic Diseases

THESE CAN be considered as external and internal. The external are mange, which has already been dealt with (see page 68) and infestation by fleas and lice. The internal are worms, of which there are the two types—round (see *Toxocara canis* infection) and tape.

External Parasitic Diseases

FLEAS

(Diagram A)

The eggs are laid on the floor or bedding and develop into adult fleas in two or three weeks.

The dog flea acts as an intermediate host for the larvae of the common tapeworm called the *Dipylidium caninum*. This

Diagram A

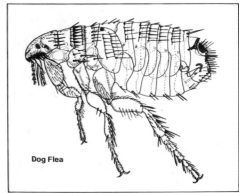

Dog Flea

makes it even more vital that flea infestation should be controlled—apart of course from the fact that dog fleas can have a good bite at the owner. In fact the human flea—the *Pulex irritans* often lives on dogs and vice versa.

Treatment and Prevention

Regular dusting, at least twice every six months, with a reputable anti-parasitic dusting powder obtained from your veterinary surgeon.

Dust the basket and bed at the same time.

A good idea is to use newspaper as a bed and burn it daily.

Modern aerosol sprays are powerful and effective *(photo 1)*.

LICE

Two species of lice occur on the dog—a suckling louse called the *Linognathus piliferous* and a biting louse called the *Trichodectes canis*. The latter, like the flea, is an

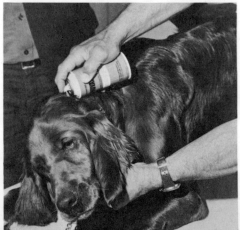

1

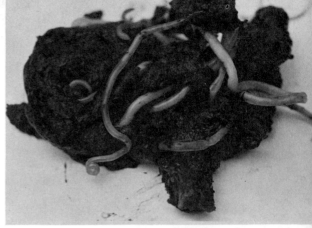

2

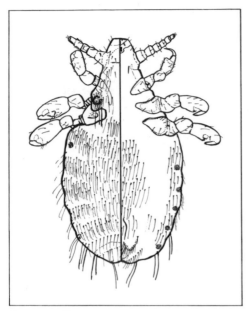

Diagram B

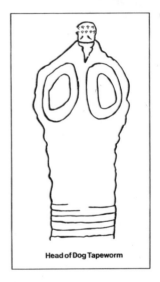

Diagram C

Head of Dog Tapeworm

intermediate host of the dog tapeworm *(Diagram B)*.

Treatment and Control
As for fleas, though in a heavy louse infestation I have found that benzene hexachloride or derris baths are most efficient and I recommend three baths at weekly intervals plus the complete destruction of all bedding.

Since the entire life cycle of the louse occurs on the dog, eradication is easier than with the flea.

Internal Parasitic Diseases
ROUNDWORM INFESTATION
There are several species of dog roundworms but the main one is the *Toxocara canis (photo 2)* which is dealt with on page 93.

The routine control of all roundworm infestation is that described for the Toxocara.

TAPEWORMS
The common tapeworm of the dog is called the *Dipylidium canium* but there are a number of others *(Diagram C)*.

The tapeworm lays its eggs in its tail segments which are shed from time to time. The eggs pass out in the dung and are eaten by the embryos of fleas and lice. Inside they develop and stay there until the flea or louse is adult.

The dog infects or re-infects itself by eating the fleas or lice.

THE TAPEWORM CANNOT DEVELOP WITHOUT AN INTERMEDIATE HOST. THIS MAKES THE ROUTINE CONTROL OF FLEAS

AND LICE ALL THE MORE IMPORT-
ANT IN YOUR DOG.

Symptoms
Since the tapeworms literally eat the dog's
food, typical signs are a voracious appetite combined with a loss in condition. The
dog will have a harsh coat and may be
markedly anaemic *(photo 2)*.

Flat segments of the tapeworm can be
seen in the motion or attached to the hairs
around the dog's anus.

Heavy infestation may cause an impaction of the intestine in which case the
dog's appetite will become capricious; he
will be uneasy and may start having fits.
Usually, however, an observant owner has
had the dog treated long before this stage
is reached.

Tapeworms occur at any age, no
apparent immunity developing as in
roundworm.

Treatment
This should be left to your veterinary
surgeon. He will always prescribe the most
effective remedy in the correct doses.

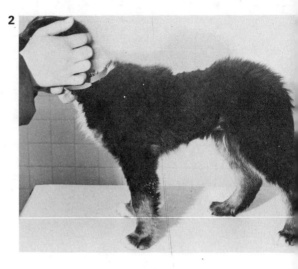

It is a good idea to take a sample of the
tapeworm segment for his inspection.

Prevention
Regular dusting against fleas and lice is in
my opinion the most valuable preventative routine in tapeworm control. Remember the tapeworm cannot develop
without an intermediary host.

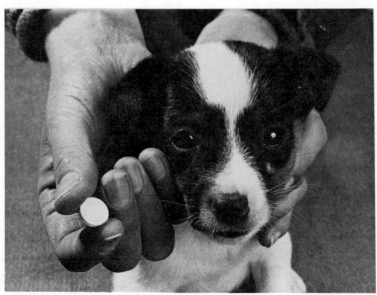

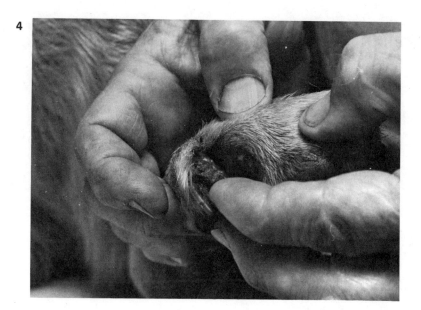

4

Subsequent Worming

It is my experience that dog owners as a whole literally have 'worms on the brain', and they ascribe countless variations in their pet's condition to the dreaded 'worms' and dose the poor creatures indiscriminately *(photo 3)*.

One simple fact to remember—over the years worming treatments have done dogs a great deal more harm than the worms themselves, so the golden rule is this—

Never dose for worms unless you see them

in the dog's motion. Then take the worm or

worms to your veterinary surgeon. He will

identify them and will prescribe the best and

safest anthelmintic.

HARVEST MITES

Not infrequently, particularly in the summer, dogs pick up between their claws so-called 'harvest mites'. They are not really mites but parasitic larvae which burrow under the skin producing a red spot in the centre of an inflamed area.

Symptoms

Extreme itching and the dog bites like mad at the affected paw or paws. The spot becomes a blister, then a scab which eventually falls off *(photo 4)*.

Treatment

Your veterinary surgeon will apply the treatment. He may use strong ammonia or one of the modern anti-parasitic aerosols; personally I prefer the latter.

LICK GRANULOMA

Sometimes secondary to the harvest mite in the paws, an infection sets up and the dog licks incessantly at the area producing what we call a lick granuloma *(photo 1, page 82)*.

Other sites for lick granulomas are the front of a foreleg or the side of a hind leg (often the hock region), that is, the areas where the dog can get at easily or comfortably.

81

F

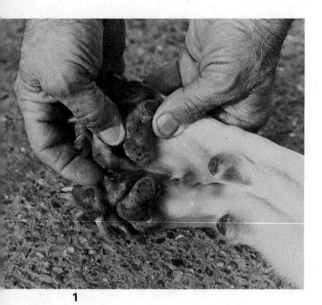

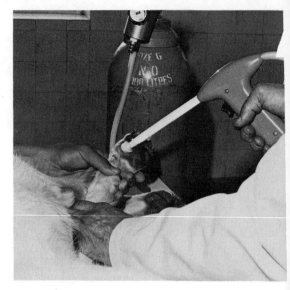

1

Cause

There seems to be a predisposition to the condition in the larger breeds, particularly the Labradors, Boxers and Great Danes.

Another contributory factor is boredom, especially when the dogs are left alone without exercise for long periods.

Treatment

Very difficult and certainly a condition for skilled veterinary attention. I have found the most satisfactory treatment to be cryosurgery *(photo 2)*, i.e., deep freezing for four or five minutes repeated in three weeks if necessary. With this therapy there is no need to bandage.

VIRUS DISEASES

24

Virus Diseases

THE MOST important of these diseases are:
1. Distemper and Hard Pad.
2. Virus Hepatitis.
3. Rabies.
4. Herpes.

Fortunately rabies is not, so far, a problem of British dogs, but it is very important in most other countries and some knowledge of the disease is desirable, especially since it may invade the country at any time.

DISTEMPER AND HARD PAD
Cause
A virus—there are various strains and the hard pad syndrome is merely associated with one of these.

Symptoms
The virus takes from one to three weeks to incubate. It then invades the entire dog's body producing a high fever and a temperature of 105°F (40·5°C) or even 106°F (41°C). This high fever lasts only for approximately 24 hours and is often missed. During the fever the virus attacks all the tissues of the body producing, in the mucous membranes particularly, minute haemorrhages.

After 24 hours the temperature returns to normal and every dog recovers from the actual virus infection (normal temp. 101.5).

Depending on the general resistance of

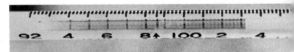

1

the dog, and especially on the standard of its feeding and environment, bacteria invade the damaged tissues and various sets of typical signs appear. When this happens the body temperature rises to between 103°F (39·5°C) and 104°F (40°C) —what we call a 'typical distemper temperature' *(photo 1)*.

When the bacteria invade the linings of the eyes and nostrils the typical signs are discharging eyes and nose *(photo 2)*. The discharge is yellowish green and the dog is dull and off its food though it may drink excessively.

2

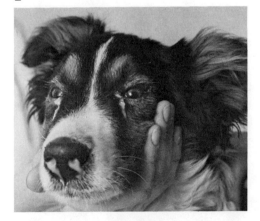

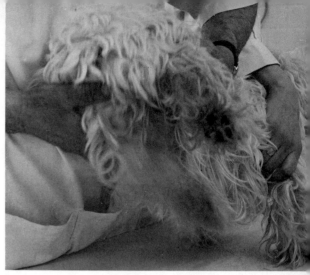

4

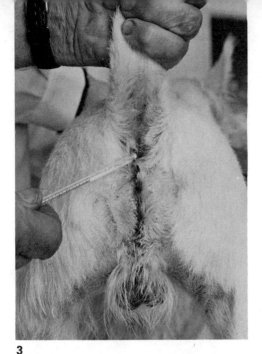

3

When the bacteria extend to the tonsils and bronchi a bronchitis develops, manifest by a harsh dry painful cough. Often it sounds as though the patient is trying to be sick. The temperature is still 103°F–(39·5°–40°C) and the dog is markedly depressed.

In some cases a broncho-pneumonia develops due simply to the bacteria multiplying in the lung tissue that was damaged by the original virus invasion. The short hacking cough gets worse, as does the filthy muco-purulent discharge from the nose which may be streaked with blood. The slightest exertion makes the dog breathe heavily—it becomes very weak and refuses all food.

When the bacteria attack the linings of the stomach and bowel—a gastro-enteritis, often acute, develops. There is incessant vomiting of a greenish or brownish mucus and a foetid diarrhoea *(photo 3)*. Often the mouth becomes ulcerated and the breath is foul. The temperature still remains at the typical 103°F–104°F (39·5°–40°C) (normal 101·5°F/38·5°C). The dog drinks water but vomits it straight back again. If he eats any food, the same thing happens.

During the diarrhoea the dog may pass worms—this is coincidental and ON NO ACCOUNT should worm medicine be given; it will make the condition very much more difficult to treat.

When organisms invade the damaged central nervous system i.e. the brain and spinal cord—nervous symptoms appear—chorea and fits which are described elsewhere. In the case illustrated, chorea produced a perpetual twitching of one hind leg *(photo 4)*. There may be a complete change of temperament—quiet dogs may become vicious; and finally paralysis usually of the hind quarters, though sometimes of the entire body. The dog becomes incontinent.

Sometimes a typical distemper rash develops on the belly and inside the thighs; the rash area is dotted over with yellow pustules *(photo 5)*.

5

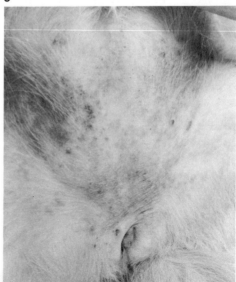

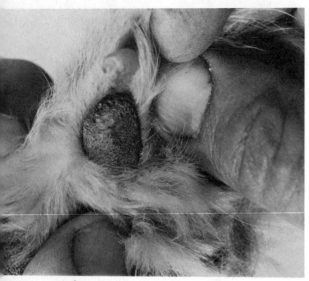

6

Immediate protection can be given to younger pups by the intramuscular injection of a measles vaccine but this lasts for a maximum of ten weeks only; during that time the correct vaccine should always be injected.

Most veterinary surgeons offer a comprehensive vaccine *(photo 7)* which in addition to protecting against distemper

7

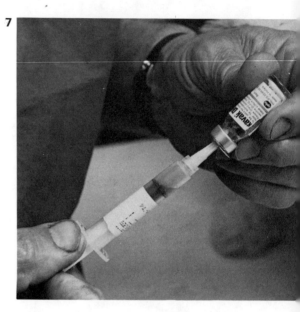

In hard pad the surfaces of the pads become thickened and hard *(photo 6)*.

These then are the typical signs of canine distemper and hard pad.

Treatment
Very much a matter for your veterinary surgeon. In my experience distemper is the most difficult and heartbreaking of all dog conditions to treat. The temperature will often persist at 103°F–104°F (39·5–40°C) for at least six weeks; then when you think you have succeeded in effecting a complete cure, chorea or fits will often start.

Prolonged courses of broad spectrum antibiotics are indicated plus eye drops, tranquillisers, etc. and weeks of intensive nursing. Without doubt it is always far cheaper to vaccinate against the disease than to have to treat it.

Prevention
Several 100 per cent vaccines are now available to everyone and NO PUP SHOULD BE LEFT WITHOUT PROTECTION.

The best age to vaccinate is nine weeks; up to that age most pups have a degree of acquired immunity from their mothers.

and hard pad affords complete immunity against the other two killer diseases, viz. leptospiral jaundice and virus hepatitis.

Two injections are needed at 14-day intervals.

Booster doses of the comprehensive vaccine should be given every one or two years.

If only every dog owner could be compelled to vaccinate, distemper and hard pad would disappear from our dog population, though the viruses could persist in foxes, ferrets, weasels and mink.

VIRUS HEPATITIS
Sometimes known as CVH (Canine Virus Hepatitis) or as Rubarth's Disease.

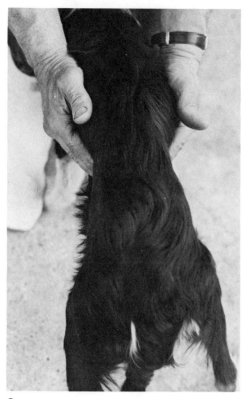

8

It can affect dogs of all ages even puppies a few days old, but usually it attacks young dogs between the ages of three and nine months.

Cause
A virus.

Symptoms
There are three types of the disease—the hyperacute, the acute and the subacute.

In the hyperacute type the dog is perfectly well in the evening and dead the next morning.

Acute cases show a high temperature up to 106°F (43·5°C) or 107°F (44·5°C) (normal 101·5°F/38·5°C). They then start typical signs of uncontrollable gastro-enteritis—vomiting and diarrhoea—which persist for nearly a week before a marked

jaundice appears. After that convulsions and death are the rule.

Subacute cases, which have comprised the majority in my experience, show a moderate fever (around 104°F) dullness and occasional vomiting. There is a well marked tenderness of the abdomen *(photo 8)*.

Often a keratitis (see 'Corneal Opacity', page 185) occurs a week or two after the start of the illness. This syndrome we call 'Blue Eye'. Occasionally, a 'Blue Eye' may appear several days after vaccination *(photo 9)*; such cases usually clear up without treatment.

I have found that if affected patients survive beyond the first week they stand a good chance of recovering completely.

Treatment
Again very much a matter for your veterinary surgeon. He will probably use a special antiserum plus vitamin K injections, in addition to treating the symptoms.

Prevention
Always vaccinate against this killer disease. Even if your dog does recover he will probably remain a carrier of the virus and a potential danger to other pups and dogs for the remainder of his life.

9

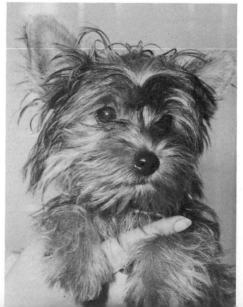

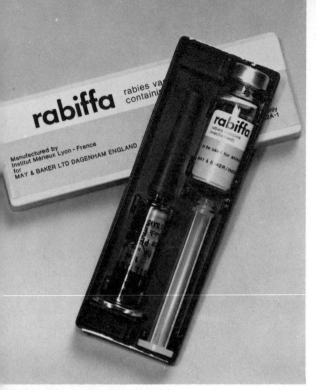

phobia, though this symptom does not appear in dogs.

3. Finally, the dog starts to stagger and eventually it falls down with its lower jaw and hind legs paralysed—this is called the 'paralysis stage'.

There is a so-called 'dumb' form of rabies in which the dog loses its bark. Such cases usually become paralysed immediately after the melancholy stage.

Treatment
Immediate euthanasia.

Prevention
In Britain, since we are free from rabies, vaccination *(photo 10)* is possible only under special licence from the Ministry of Agriculture and such licences are issued only for dogs that are going abroad.

10

RABIES

Sometimes known as hydrophobia. It is an acutely dangerous disease that can kill humans as well as practically all other mammals. In fact rabies is nearly always fatal in man.

Cause
A virus which is present in the saliva of infected dogs.

Symptoms
There are three stages in the dog:

1. A stage of acute dullness called the 'melancholy stage' during which there is a complete change in the dog's temperament. Nervous dogs become quiet and easy-going dogs become restless.

2. 'The excitement stage'. The patient becomes markedly excited and disregards his food or bolts it wildly. Later he will eat or chew at anything—straw, stones, wood etc. If locked in a kennel he will bite his way out and when free he'll bite anything in his path, (the 'mad dog' syndrome). If he bites a human, the human develops a fear of water—hence the name hydro-

HERPES AND 'FADING'

Cause
A virus.

Symptoms
The canine herpes virus causes what is

11

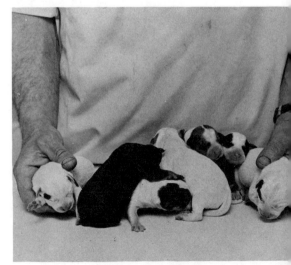

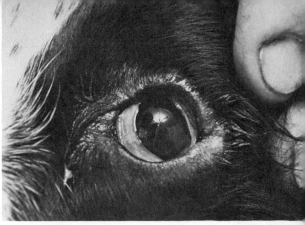

12

called 'fading' in puppies *(photo 11)*. The pups become progressively weaker despite an abundance of milk in the mother. They stop sucking, start 'paddling' and die; sometimes the bitch kills them.

Other causes of 'fading' are canine virus hepatitis, a blood incompatibility similar to that occurring in humans, and perhaps the most frequent cause of all hypothermia or 'chilling' (see 'Whelping', page 39). Another cause of fading is a germ called the *Brucella bronchiseptica* which causes the respiratory complications in distemper.

A herpes virus occasionally causes blisters on the penis, sheath and testicles of a dog. This could be a source of the 'fading' problem.

A mild form of herpes virus is thought to cause irritating bare patches to appear round a dog's eye or eyes *(photo 12)* and occasionally on the nostrils and chin. The dog scratches the eye and produces a secondary conjunctivitis. Similar lesions can appear on owners usually around the mouth.

Treatment

There is none for the acute herpes infection which hits puppies.

The mild eye, nose and chin infections, however, rapidly respond to a daily application of chloramphenicol ointment—a 10–14 day course will clear up most cases *(photo 13)*.

13

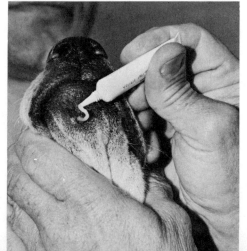

PAROVIRUS INFECTION
This is a comparatively new canine infection which has appeared since 1978.

Cause
A Canine Parovirus which in many ways is identical to the virus that causes feline (cat) enteritis.

Symptoms
A severe and often fatal gastro-enteritis which affects chiefly young, recently-weaned pups, but it can also hit older animals.

The temperature is usually normal or subnormal and the faeces may be blood stained.

In very young pups, the virus damages the heart muscle and produces death from heart failure.

Treatment
Skilled veterinary attention is vital. Death is often due to severe dehydration, which the veterinary surgeon can combat with oral and intravenous fluid therapy. At the same time he will prescribe broad-spectrum antibiotics to control secondary bacteria.

Prevention
Some protection can be given by using the cat vaccine against feline enteritis. I feel sure a satisfactory canine vaccine will soon be produced by the scientists.

25

Leptospirosis

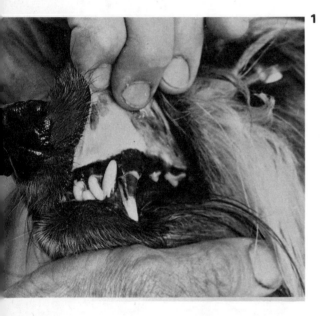

1 THIS DISEASE is known as leptospiral jaundice or infectious jaundice.

Cause
An organism called a spirochaete with the rather complicated name of *Leptospira icterohaemorrhagiae*. This spirochaete causes a serious disease in man called Weil's Disease and is carried by nearly half of the rat population.

Dogs become infected by eating food that has been contaminated by rat urine or by eating infected rats.

When a dog or a human is infected the spirochaete passes out in the urine.

Symptoms
The dog goes off its food, vomits and lies about miserably.

On examination the membranes of the eye and the mouth are seen to have the typical yellow tinge of jaundice *(photo 1)*.

2 The jaundice rapidly worsens and the eyes and mouth become bright yellow or golden.

The patient becomes tucked up and rapidly loses condition. He shows clear signs of pain when the abdomen is pressed *(photo 2)*.

The dung is dark and foul smelling, thick at first but rapidly becoming diarrhoeic.

Within the first 48 hours or so the temperature is high—up to 105°F (40·5°C) or 106°F (41°C) but it drops down to subnormal.

Treatment

This is a very difficult condition to treat and the prognosis is bad unless caught early.

The veterinary surgeon will inject antiserum and antibiotics. Advanced cases will require fluid injection therapy and fanatical nursing.

Prevention

Obviously it is the duty of every pet owner to protect his animal against this evil disease. It can be done simply by insisting that the vaccination of the pup and subsequent boosters is a comprehensive one providing complete cover against distemper, hard pad, leptospirosis and virus hepatitis.

LEPTOSPIRA CANICOLA INFECTION

Sometimes known as Stuttgart Disease.

Cause

A less virulent spirochaete called the *Leptospira canicola*.

Symptoms

These vary from acute symptoms to those described for nephritis (see 'Nephritis', page 171).

When the *Leptospira canicola* invades the bloodstream the patient runs a temperature of around 104°F and goes off its food. There is a pronounced thirst; the dog starts to vomit and there is a foul smell from the breath *(photo 3)*. Jaundice may but usually doesn't appear. The temperature drops to normal after two days and ulcers may develop on the tongue.

These symptoms are due largely to the kidney damage that the *Leptospira canicola* produces.

Mild canicola infections are often manifest as nephritis.

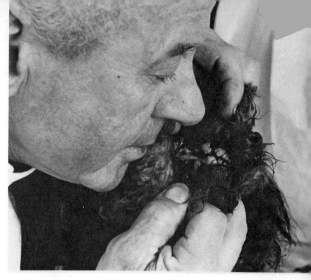

3

Treatment

If the case is caught early, it responds extremely well to massive doses of penicillin.

Once the kidneys are badly damaged, however, a nephritis becomes established which is very much more difficult to treat.

Stuttgart Disease describes advanced cases where the mouth is covered with evil-smelling ulcers *(photo 4)* and vomiting is uncontrollable. It is my experience that such cases invariably die.

Prevention

The Leptospira vaccines contain antibodies against the canicola as well as the icterohaemorrhagiae and provide a full and efficient protection—so vaccinate your pup at nine and eleven weeks and make sure he has a booster vaccination at least every two years.

4

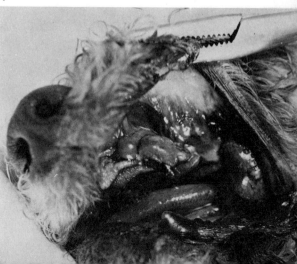

26
Diseases Dangerous to Humans

APART FROM ringworm and herpes (see 'Ringworm', page 71) and 'Herpes', page 88), there are only two, neither of which could be regarded as more than remotely dangerous, and one of which is just as likely to be transferred from humans to dogs. Occasional Press panic, therefore, about the danger of keeping pets is absolute nonsense *(photo 1)*.

TOXOPLASMOSIS
Cause
A single-celled parasite called the *Toxoplasma gondii* which can be carried by

man, cattle, sheep, pigs, rabbits and birds as well as by dogs. The parasite can cause defective eyesight or blindness in humans.

Symptoms
In dogs toxoplasmosis flares up as a complication of distemper. It produces encephalitis or inflammation of the brain leading to abnormal behaviour, convulsions, paralysis and death *(photo 2)*.

Treatment
There is none.

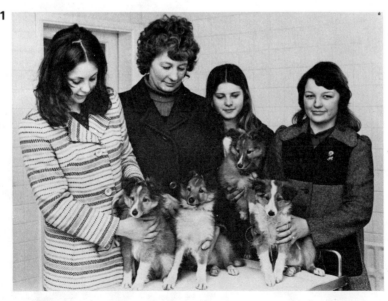

92

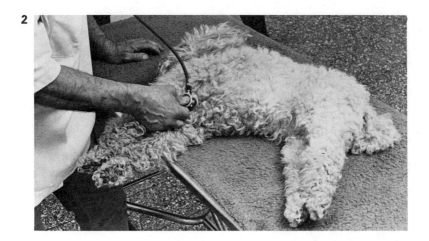

Danger to Humans

Almost negligible. Recorded cases are few and far between and even in these it has never been fully established that the dog gave the disease to the humans or vice versa.

TOXOCARA CANIS INFECTION

This is more dangerous especially to children, and the following observations should be studied very carefully by all pet-owners.

Cause

The larva or intermediate stage of a common roundworm found particularly in whelping bitches and pups. The worm is called the *Toxocara canis (photo 3)*.

The roundworm lays sticky eggs which pass out in the faeces of the pups and stick to the hairs of their coats or to the whelping box or bedding.

If a child handles the bitch or puppies, some of the eggs may stick to the skin

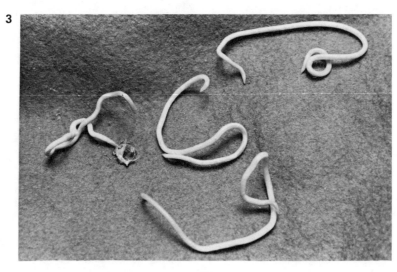

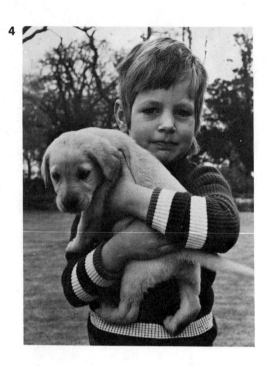

4

geon; he will prescribe the most effective drug. DOSE EXACTLY ACCORDING TO HIS INSTRUCTIONS.

When breeding, dose the bitch for roundworms during the first week of pregnancy.

If you purchase a pup of any age, always seek your veterinary surgeon's advice regarding roundworm dosing, regardless of what the breeder has done.

Danger to Humans
Obviously the danger does exist but it is absolutely minimal and a simple adherence to the above routine will eliminate it altogether.

Incidentally, the roundworm of cats called the *Toxocara cati* provides a similar hazard and cats should be dosed for roundworms every six months.

In addition, children should be taught to wash their hands thoroughly after handling their pets.

(photo 4). There they develop into larvae which pierce the skin and migrate through the child's body. Practically all of the larvae die, but just occasionally (no more than once in a million infections) the larvae reach the back of the child's eye and cause defective vision or even blindness.

Toxocara canis is chiefly a parasite of the younger puppy. It is passed from the mother into the pup before it is born.

It arrives in the pup's intestine three days after birth and grows into an adult worm in six days.

EGG PRODUCTION BEGINS WHEN THE PUP IS ABOUT TWO MONTHS OLD. THE ADULT WORM VIRTUALLY DISAPPEARS FROM DOGS OVER TWELVE MONTHS OLD.

Prevention
Conscientiously dose all pups for roundworms at six weeks, eight weeks, four months and eight months *(photo 5)*. Get the worm tablets from a veterinary sur-

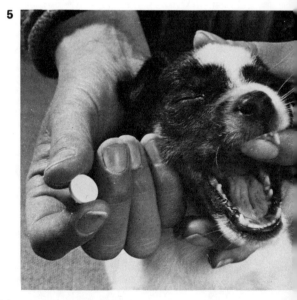

5

GENERAL DISEASES AND CONDITIONS

27
The Bones

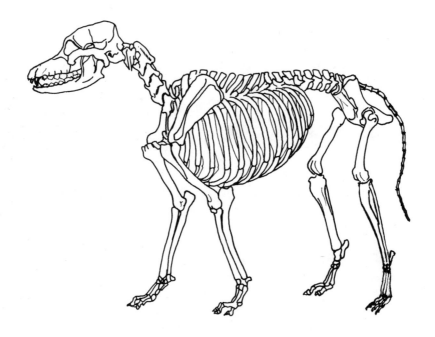

THERE ARE a number of complicated bone diseases but most are rare and require highly skilled scientific knowledge to treat, e.g. osteomalacia and osteo-distrophia. Obviously, therefore, it is sensible to deal only with the simple and common conditions. They are:

1. Fractures.
2. Arthritis.
3. Rickets.
4. Tumours.
5. Ostitis.
6. Periostitis.
7. Disc Displacement and Paralysis.
8. Docking and Dew Claws.

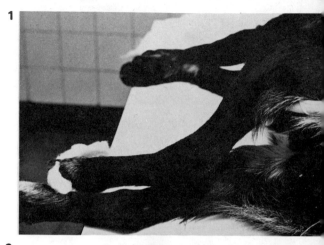

FRACTURES

In every veterinary practice bone fractures in the dog are a daily occurrence *(photo 1)*. In fact I would say they occur so frequently that many of our veterinary surgeons are as skilled in orthopaedics (bone surgery) as their human counterparts.

Cause

By and large, road accidents. The ever-increasing weight of traffic and the inevitable straying dogs provide a continuous flow of cases.

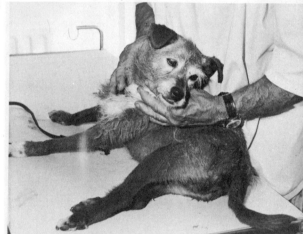

Treatment

Every suspect fracture case should be taken immediately to a veterinary surgeon *(photo 2)*.

By using his experience and X-rays he will decide exactly what to do.

Depending on the site and type of fracture he will splint it *(photo 3)*, plaster it or admit it to hospital.

Many modern veterinary hospitals are as good as or even better than human ones.

The clinic illustrated for example is the personal property of the author and many small animal owners have genuinely stated they would rather bring their children here than take them to hospital. I laughingly point out that the intensive care pens are scarcely big enough for that purpose.

Continued on page 99

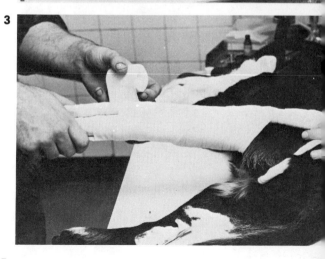

97

G

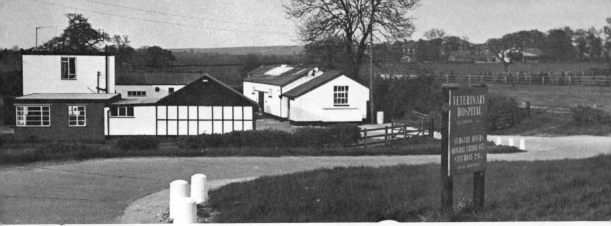

Veterinary Hospital

1. General view of the author's modern hospital.
2. Waiting Room. 3. Operating Theatre.
4. Consulting Room. 5 and 6. The Intensive
Care Unit.

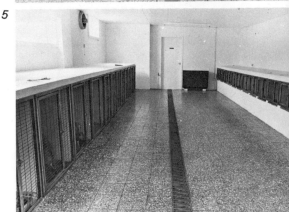

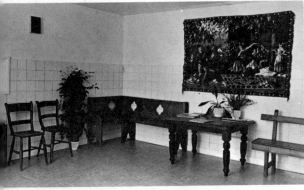

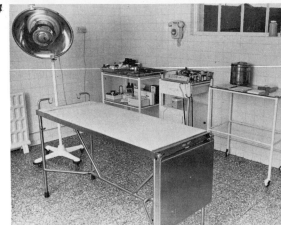

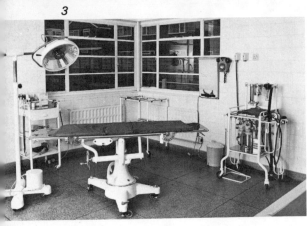

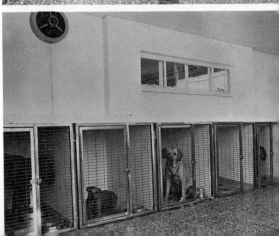

98

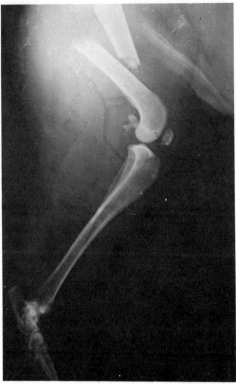

4

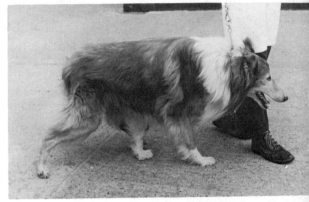

ARTHRITIS
Arthritis simply means inflammation of the joints and this inflammation makes walking an effort *(photo 5)*.

Cause
In dogs it may or may not be associated with rheumatism. I see it most often in older dogs where there is usually a history of injury to the affected limb. The hip joint is often involved.

Symptoms
Intermittent or persistent stiffness or marked lameness, and difficulty in rising *(photo 6)*.

Pain is evinced when the affected joint is manipulated.

Positive diagnosis requires X-ray evidence.

ORTHOPAEDIC SURGERY
Bone-pinning, plating, transplants and all other aspects of orthopaedic surgery are now practised on dogs. This means that practically any fracture no matter how severe and complicated can be repaired.

Perhaps one of the most frequent canine orthopaedic operations is the bone pinning or plating of a fractured femur *(photo 4)*, a bone often broken in car accidents. The series of photographs on page 100 illustrate the highly successful technique usually employed. It is easier to illustrate a plating than a pinning.

Orthopaedic surgery is expensive but, for the sake of the dog, most veterinary surgeons will do everything possible to keep the cost within the pocket of the owner.

6

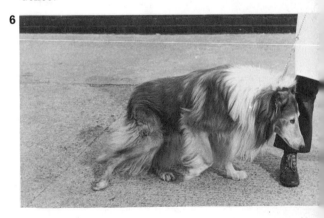

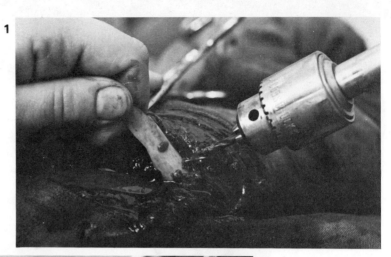

Plating a Fractured Femur

Three stages in
the technique referred
to on page 99
(under 'Orthopaedic
Surgery').

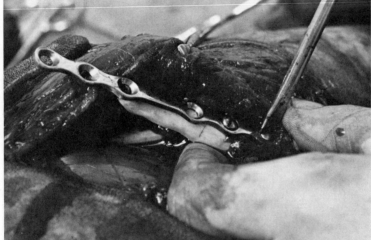

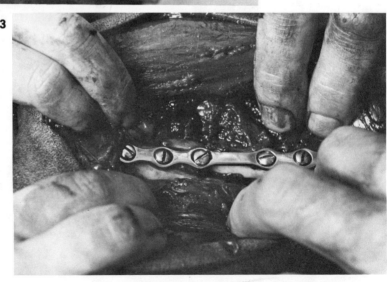

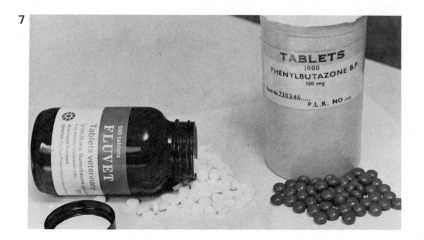

7

Treatment
Intermittent or prolonged courses of cortisone and butazoladin, though the results are variable and rarely completely successful *(photo 7)*.

Hip arthritis may be alleviated or cured by orthopaedic surgery.

RICKETS
Seen in puppies, but because of general improvement in nutrition, nothing like as common as it used to be.

Cause
Aphosphorosis, i.e. a deficiency of the mineral phosphorus. This can be triggered off by a lack of vitamin D or phosphorus or a shortage of both.

Symptoms
Enlarged ends of the long bones and a bending of the shafts; in other words, the pups become knock-kneed or bowlegged *(photo 8)*.

Lumps form at the bottom of each rib bone where it joins its cartilage about two-thirds of the way down the chest.

If untreated, rachitic pups rapidly lose

condition, have a capricious appetite and develop diarrhoea and a 'pot-belly'.

Treatment
One halibut liver oil capsule daily plus one teaspoonful of bone meal well mixed up in the food. The halibut liver oil provides

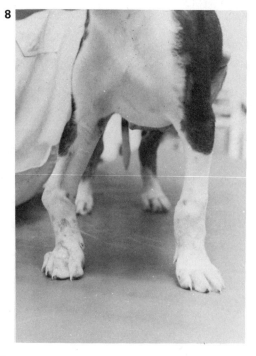

8

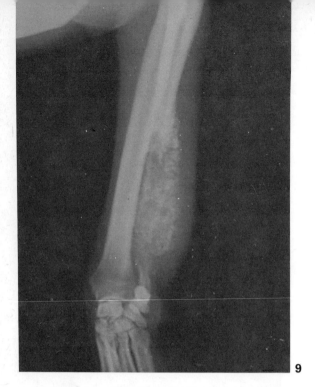
9

TUMOURS: CANCER OF THE BONE

Cancer of the bone called osteosarcoma is not uncommon in dogs. It occurs chiefly in the leg bones where the bone cells are invaded by the tumour *(photo 9)*. Occasionally it is seen in the bones of the head.

Symptoms
The first sign is usually lameness. The part affected is thickened to twice or even three times its normal size. If neglected, the bone will bend or break. When the skull is affected, the bone becomes a pulpy mess.

Treatment
Immediate amputation where a leg bone is involved *(photo 10)*.

Prognosis
Must be guarded; secondary osteo-sarcomas are liable to develop elsewhere but amputation can sometimes prolong life for two or three years or even longer. The patient illustrated, for example, is a working farm dog and was operated on $4\frac{1}{2}$ years ago.

the essential vitamin D and the bone meal the phosphorus. If yeast tablets are being given, stop them until the condition is clear.

Do Ricket Cases Recover?
Yes, completely—provided the treatment is started reasonably early, any undue delay leads to permanent leg disfiguration.

10

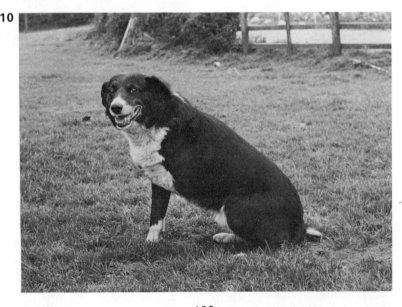

OSTITIS
Simply means inflammation of the bone.

Cause
Injury or infection—sometimes secondary to orthopaedic surgery.

Symptoms
Acute lameness and pain; if infection is present, the temperature rises to 106°F (41°C). There is marked swelling.

Treatment
If due to injury and no fever is present, rest and patience are all that are required.

If infection is present, blitz treatment with a prolonged course of broad spectrum antibiotics is necessary.

PERIOSTITIS
Means inflammation of the periosteum, which is the membrane covering all bones. It invariably occurs at the same time as ostitis and its symptoms and treatment are identical.

DISC DISPLACEMENT AND PARALYSIS
This is seen chiefly in long-backed dogs such as Dachshunds *(photo 11)* and Bassets, though it can occur in any breed.

11

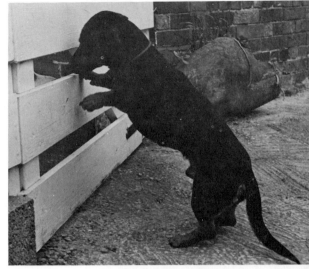

12

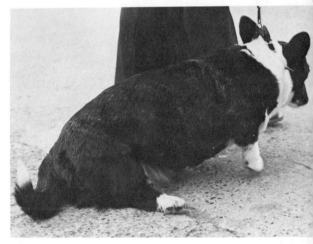

13

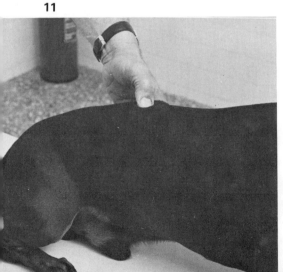

Cause
Rapid twisting or turning during violent exercise or attempted jumping of high fences *(photo 12)*.

Symptoms
Partial or complete loss of control of the hind quarters *(photo 13)*. Considerable pain may be evinced when the spine is handled.

103

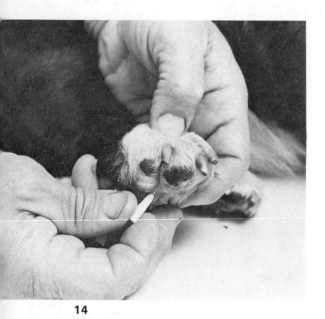

14

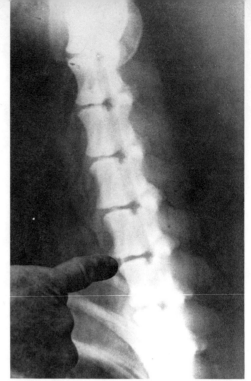

16

Where the paralysis is complete, the reflexes may disappear from the hind legs *(photo 14)*.

Diagnosis is confirmed by X-ray *(photos 15 and 16)*.

Treatment
Very much a matter for the veterinary surgeon though considerable patience and co-operation will be required of the owner, especially if the paralysis is complete.

15

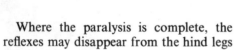

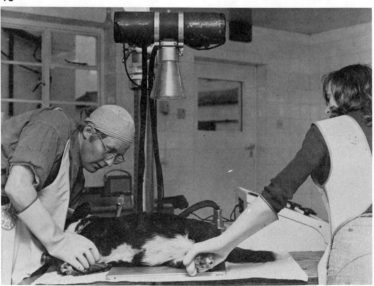

It is my experience that cases which can stand, no matter how groggily, have the best chance of recovery. In such animals the displacement is only partial.

Treatment comprises manipulation under a general anaesthetic followed by a prolonged course of steroids and/or pain killers, e.g. a hormone called nandrolone.

In the partial displacements a protective capsule of fibrous tissue forms round the disc protruberance and the dog eventually goes reasonably sound.

Where paralysis is complete, the prognosis is bad and euthanasia should always be considered.

OTHER CAUSES OF PARALYSIS

These may be a stroke (see 'Cerebral Haemorrhage', page 198, spinal haemorrhage or fracture secondary to injury, osteosarcoma of the spine (see 'Osteosarcoma', page 102), nervous sequelae of distemper (see 'Distemper), and a fractured pelvis *(photo 17)*. The diagnosis and treatment of all these should be left to your veterinary surgeon.

A fractured pelvis in a dog often heals remarkably well.

The sole treatment required in many

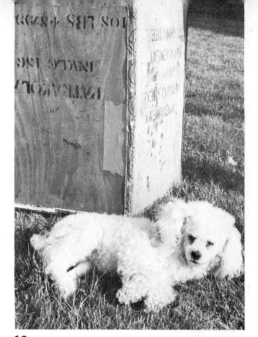

18

cases is to confine the dog to a restricted space (a large tea chest suits admirably) for a month or six weeks; lifting the dog out onto the grass two or three times a day to empty his bladder and bowels *(photo 18)*.

DOCKING

Removing the tails from puppies is in the process of being made illegal in Britain *(photo 19)*. I think this is a good thing because such mutilation has been performed only to satisfy fashion and vanity.

The docking of adult tails, however, by veterinary surgeons, will still be permissable under general anaesthesia but only for justifiable surgical reasons.

17

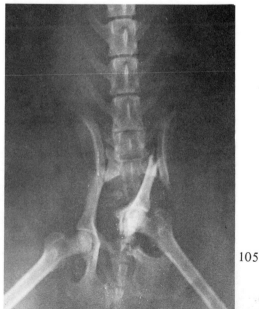

19

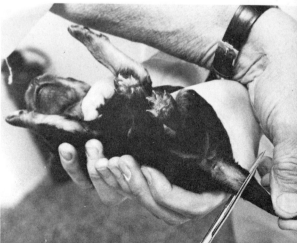

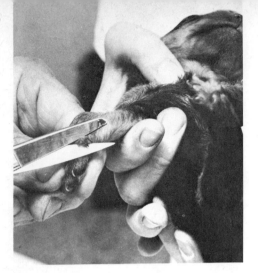

20

THE REMOVAL OF DEW CLAWS

This is a practical and sensible operation *(photo 20)*. The best age to perform it is when pups are seven days old. It should be done by a veterinary surgeon, who will

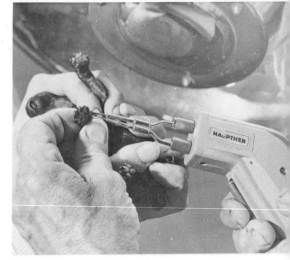

21

take the proper steps to control haemorrhage and infection *(photo 21)*.

28
Congenital or Hereditary Defects

The Hip *(Diagram A)*

UNFORTUNATELY IN many pedigree breeds there has been a great deal of indiscriminate in-breeding and this has led to a disturbing increase in the number of congenital defects.

It is my opinion that the days of the present pedigree breeds are numbered. It is only a matter of time before dog breeders follow the lead of the breeders of all other classes of stock (horses, cattle, sheep and pigs) and go in for selected cross-breeding to produce hybrid vigour. Until this is done I'm afraid we shall have to face an ever-increasing number of hereditary diseases.

Diagram A

NORMAL ANATOMY OF HIP JOINT

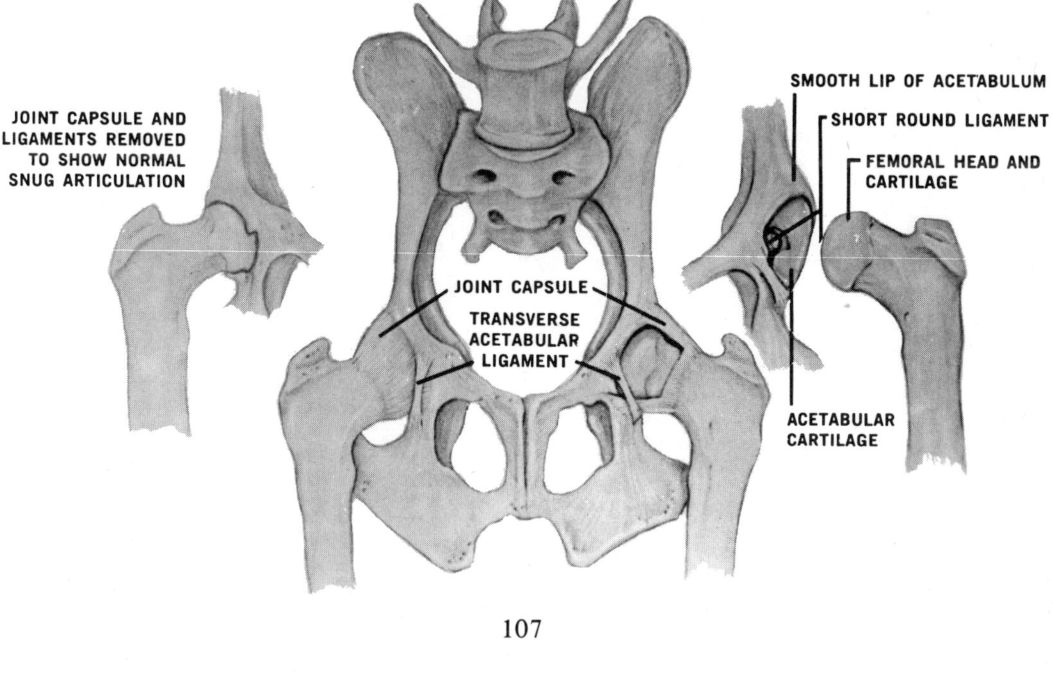

JOINT CAPSULE AND LIGAMENTS REMOVED TO SHOW NORMAL SNUG ARTICULATION

SMOOTH LIP OF ACETABULUM

SHORT ROUND LIGAMENT

FEMORAL HEAD AND CARTILAGE

JOINT CAPSULE

TRANSVERSE ACETABULAR LIGAMENT

ACETABULAR CARTILAGE

Perhaps the commonest now occurring in practically all breeds is:

HIP DYSPLASIA

This is a condition where the head of the femur or main thigh bone is abnormal and does not fit into the acetabulum or hip socket properly *(see diagram B)*.

There are a number of varying types of dysplasia which require skilled veterinary X-ray diagnosis to distinguish, but the symptoms are very similar.

Symptoms

The first sign—seen mainly in Alsatians *(photo 1)*, Golden Labradors and Boxers —is a reluctance to rise from the sitting position and a sawing or unsteady gait first observed when the pup is four to six months old. Thereafter as the dog's weight increases, the condition tends to get progressively worse *(photo 2)*.

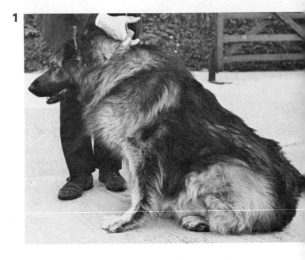

1

Treatment

The diagnosis and treatment should be left entirely to the veterinary surgeon *(photo 3)*.

One type, called Perthe's disease, may clear up spontaneously within six months.

Diagram B

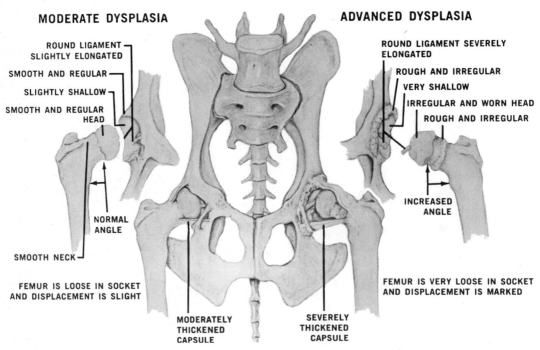

MODERATE DYSPLASIA

ROUND LIGAMENT SLIGHTLY ELONGATED

SMOOTH AND REGULAR

SLIGHTLY SHALLOW

SMOOTH AND REGULAR HEAD

NORMAL ANGLE

SMOOTH NECK

FEMUR IS LOOSE IN SOCKET AND DISPLACEMENT IS SLIGHT

MODERATELY THICKENED CAPSULE

SEVERELY THICKENED CAPSULE

ADVANCED DYSPLASIA

ROUND LIGAMENT SEVERELY ELONGATED

ROUGH AND IRREGULAR

VERY SHALLOW

IRREGULAR AND WORN HEAD

ROUGH AND IRREGULAR

INCREASED ANGLE

FEMUR IS VERY LOOSE IN SOCKET AND DISPLACEMENT IS MARKED

108

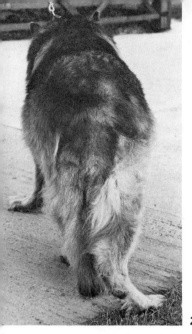

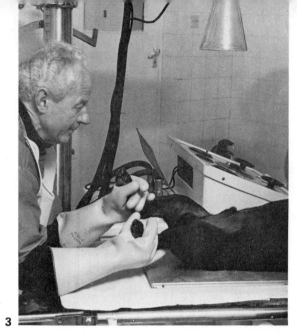

2   3

Some of the other types may respond to drastic orthopaedic surgery comprising removal of the head of the femur, but at all times diagnosis and treatment should be left entirely to your veterinary surgeon.

Many cases in young dogs respond to an operation called pectineal myotomy, which involves cutting the pectineal muscle on one or both sides of the inner thigh *(photos 4, 5 and 6)*.

By no means are all hip dysplasia conditions hopeless. Slight cases may live out a useful life span without surgery, though the weakness may always be apparent particularly after exercise.

Many others can be alleviated by orthopaedic surgery.

Never, under any circumstances, should bitches or dogs suffering from dysplasia be used for breeding. In fact, if breeding for show or sale it is wise to have both bitches and stud dogs cleared by X-ray before service.

The Stifle

LUXATING PATELLA

Another equally common hereditary defect is luxation or dislocation of the

5

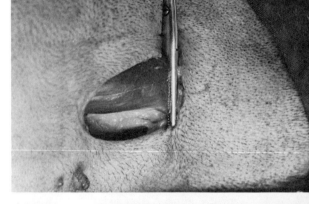

4

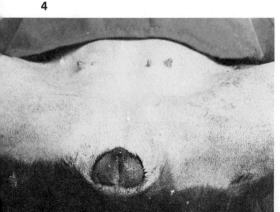

6

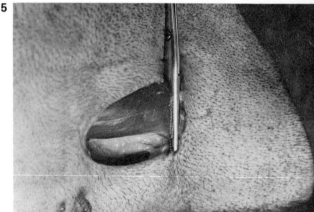

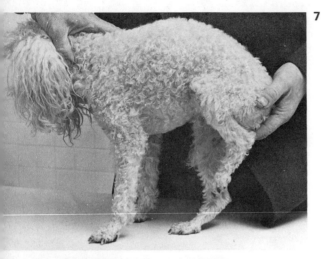

7

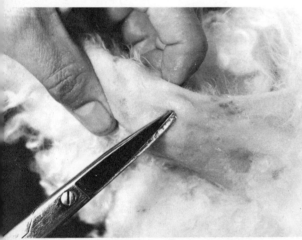

8

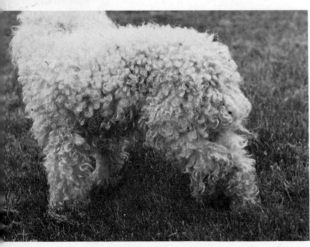

9

patella or knee-cap which is situated in the dog's stifle joint *(photo 7)*. In my experience this occurs most frequently in the smaller breeds—pedigree Poodles, Terriers, Griffons, Pekes, Pomeranians, Papillons and Chihuahuas, though I have seen it in Boxers, Bulldogs and Labradors.

In luxation of the patella one or other of the ligaments which hold it in position *(photo 8)*—usually the anterior cruciate ligament is torn or irreparably damaged and the patella keeps slipping in and out of position. Sometimes both stifles are involved.

Symptoms
Intermittent or persistent hind leg lameness *(photo 9)*. The patient may return from exercise on three legs and may or may not exhibit acute pain. On manipulating the stifle joint and straightening the hind leg, the patella can be felt clicking into position.

Treatment
Very much a matter for the veterinary surgeon.

In mild cases particularly where both stifles are involved, false joints are formed after a time and apparent lameness disappears.

Where the lameness and luxation are persistently acute, and especially when the dog refuses to use the leg, then orthopaedic surgery is required and the sooner it is embarked upon the greater the chance of complete success *(photo 10)*.

The operation comprises tendon splitting and fixation of the patella in its correct position and is completely successful in many cases. Sometimes the patella has to be drilled and wired into position *(photo 11)*.

Prevention
The only hope for the future lies in selective cross-breeding.

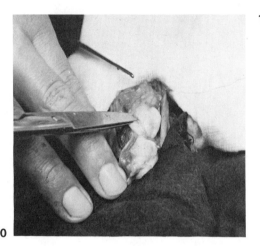

10

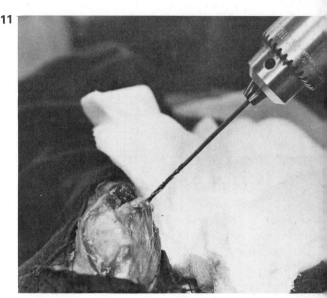

11

RETINAL ATROPHY

The retina is the innermost and light-sensitive coat of the posterior part of the globe of the eye *(photo 12)* (see 'The Eye'). Atrophy simply means wasting, and in retinal atrophy the retina is imperfectly developed and usually continues to waste or shrivel up. I have seen the condition particularly in Red Setters and Poodles.

Symptoms

The first sign is usually an apparent inability to see in the dark (night blindness). The dog will run into objects when taken out at night.

Treatment

There is none. The condition tends to progressively worsen and leads to permanent blindness.

Prevention

The only hope for the elimination of congenital retinal atrophy is selective cross-breeding. No amount of legislation is likely to succeed in controlling close breeding.

CONGENITAL CATARACT

Cataract (see 'The Eye', page 188) is an opacity or clouding of the crystalline lens

of the eye. Usually both lenses are affected.

Normally this occurs only in ageing dogs.

Symptoms

In congenital cataract the signs are seen early—within hours of purchasing an affected pup it will be seen to run into objects. The veterinary surgeon will be

12

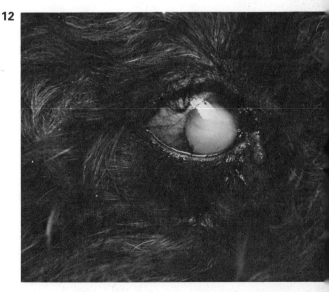

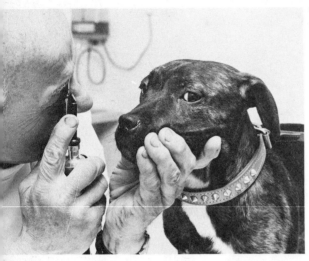

able to diagnose the condition quickly by examining the eye with an opthalmoscope *(photo 13)*.

Treatment
So far there is none, though at the moment I am privately researching into the removal of the affected lenses combined with the experimental fitting of the new soft lens contact lenses. Such experiments

are needless to say expensive but at least hold out some hope for the future.

Prevention
Cessation of in-breeding or, better still, selective cross-breeding.

DEAFNESS

This occurs frequently in white Bull Terriers but I have seen it in Terriers and Poodles *(photo 14)*.

Treatment
There is none though the affected dog can learn to live very happily in his or her own familiar environment. The danger lies with traffic; if allowed off the lead near a road, a deaf dog is much more liable to be run over than a normal one.

Prevention
It is doubtful whether selective cross-breeding would eliminate congenital deafness. In white dogs particularly it seems to be associated with the albino or white colouring rather than in-breeding.

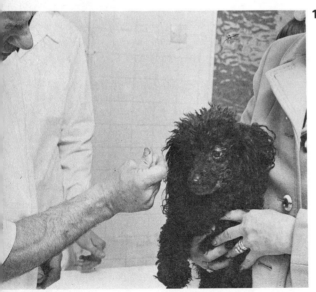

14

HARE-LIP

Hare-lip is a malformation of the upper lip where the two halves are separated sometimes widely *(photo 15)*.
I have seen it in Bulldog pups and in several of the toy breeds.

Symptoms
Obvious and rapid wasting in the pup since sucking with the hare-lip is difficult or impossible. Even mild cases do not thrive as they should.

Treatment
Surgery is successful only occasionally because the hare-lip condition is often

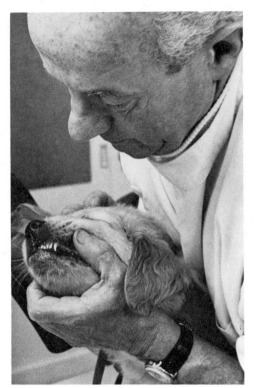

15

associated with a 'cleft palate''.

CLEFT PALATE

This is a hereditary defect of the roof of
the mouth generally seen in in-bred pups
of the toy breeds.

There is a gap in the structures forming
the palate.

Symptoms
Usually a dead or unthrifty pup since the
cleft palate makes sucking impossible or
at best extremely difficult.

Treatment
In my opinion it is wise to cull such pups
immediately. Surgery is not only un-
economical but rarely successful.

Prevention
Avoid in-breeding.

HERNIAS
Probably the most common cogenital
hernia is the unbilical *(photo 16)* (see
'Umbilical Hernia', page 30).

Another form, seen in well-bred bitches,
is the inguinal hernia seen in the inguinal
region at the top of the inside of the hind
leg *(photo 17)*.

16
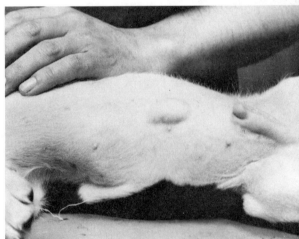

17
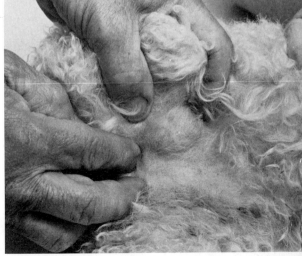

113

29
The Muscles

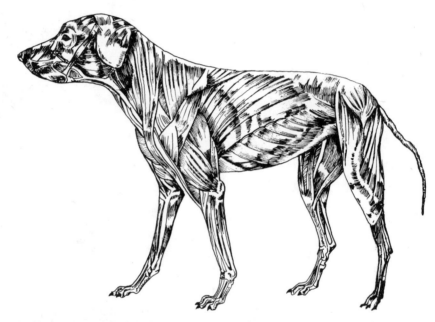

THE MUSCLES of the dog are extremely well developed and under natural conditions muscular troubles would be rare. However, for various reasons they occur frequently among domestic pets.

FIBROSITIS

This is by far the most common muscular condition we have to deal with. The term fibrositis simply means inflammation of the muscle fibres.

Cause

Exposure to draughts, cold or wet parti-

cularly after being kept in over-heated houses.

The crazy habit of clipping Poodles in mid-winter is in my experience, the most frequent predisposing cause *(photo 1)*. Often a poor little shivering Poodle is brought to me screaming its head off with

1

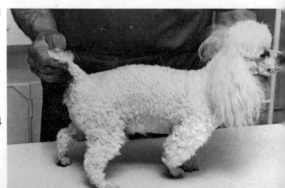

114

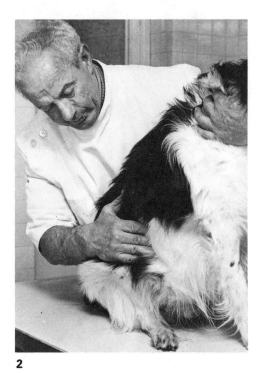

2

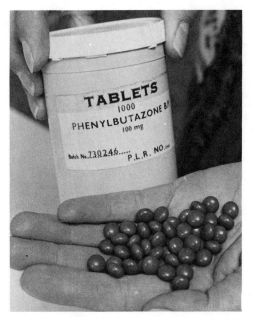

3

fibrositis. When I bluntly tell the owner how stupid they are, they become quite indignant. As an old veterinary surgeon I worked for used to say, "There's no medicine in the world that can cure a fool". How right he was!

Symptoms
Acute muscular pain; intermittently the dog will scream out when touched or picked up. The pain seems to move from one muscular region to another.

Examination shows groups of muscles to be tensed up, hard and painful *(photo 2)*.

Dogs of any age can be affected. I have seen a litter of pups with it when only six weeks old.

Treatment
The veterinary surgeon will inject long-acting cortisone which will afford rapid relief. He will then follow that up with a seven-to-ten-day course of a drug called butazoladin which acts efficiently against all muscular and joint pains *(photo 3)*. The old fashioned aspirin tablets provide a good first-aid treatment. The dose? One to four depending on size.

Clipped Poodles should be provided with a woollen or fur coat which covers the loins *(photo 4)*. Owners should be told

4

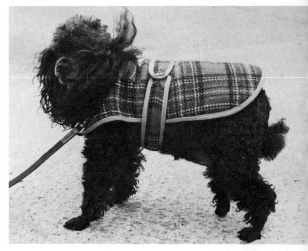

115

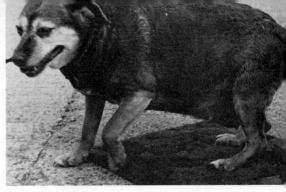

clearly that clipping should be done only in the warm summer weather; I always tell the Poodle fans that the time to clip is when the farmer clips his sheep.

Affected working dogs should be kept out of water.

Prognosis
Very good, though the condition will recur unless care is taken.

MUSCULAR RHEUMATISM

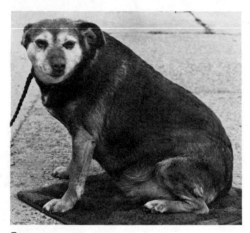

5

Seen mostly in older dogs *(photo 5)*.

Cause
The predisposing causes are the same as for fibrositis but often, as in older humans, lack of exercise, plus senility seem the chief factors.

Symptoms
Difficulty in rising and stiffness especially first thing in the morning *(photo 6)*. The symptoms improve or disappear as the day wears on.

Pain may not be apparent during examination, though the muscles feel unnaturally tensed.

Treatment
As for fibrositis, though cortisone may be

6

contra-indicated if the heart is suspect. Obviously treatment should be carried out under veterinary supervision.

Once again, aspirin is a safe first-aid treatment.

MUSCULAR DYSTROPHY

A condition where the muscles waste and don't function properly. It is not common in dogs but I have seen it in Greyhounds *(photo 7)*.

Cause
Not absolutely clear but is associated with deficiency of vitamin E. The outbreak in Greyhounds I helped to investigate proved to be due to the exclusive feeding of food that had been boiled.

Symptoms
Loss of muscular condition—death due to heart failure.

The affected Greyhounds were dropping dead during races.

Treatment
Injections and oral administration of vitamin E.

7

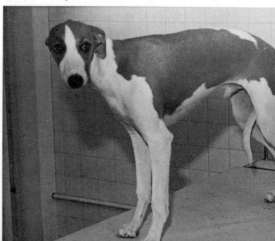

Prevention
Always feed a percentage of unboiled food, especially raw green vegetables, in the diet.

MUSCULAR CRAMP
It is my experience that this condition occurs chiefly in Scottish Terriers *(photo 8)*. I have seen it in other breeds, especially town dogs that are suddenly given access to the wide open spaces of the country.

Cause
Work or exercise when the muscles are not in a fit condition.

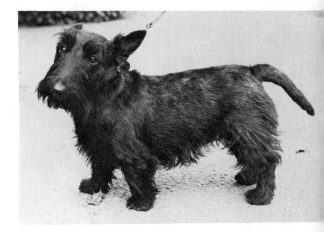

8

Symptoms
In Scotties, usually the younger ones up to two years old, the typical signs are— they will set off at a brisk trot or run then after about two or three hundred yards or even less they will stop and collapse, or squeal out in pain. The muscles are tensed and hard as in fibrositis but the condition is more generalised and after a few minutes the spasm will disappear.

Sometimes, in mild cases, the only sign is a difficulty in getting up the steps into the house after a walk.

Treatment
The veterinary surgeon may prescribe calcium or parathyroid therapy, but the attacks seem to disappear as the terrier gets older.

The old-fashioned remedy of a pinch of salt daily in the food is well worth trying.

Prevention
'Scottie cramp' could, in my opinion, be eliminated by the avoidance of in-breeding or by selective cross-breeding.

30
Common Disorders of the Mouth

FOREIGN BODY
Symptoms
The dog slobbers profusely *(photo 1)* and is unable to eat. Examination of the mouth shows either a piece of bone or stick stuck across the roof of the mouth or between the teeth.

Treatment
Quite simple: remove it *(photo 2)*—but this is often a job for a veterinary surgeon as the dog is usually in some pain and distress.

HAEMORRHAGE
Symptoms
Bleeding is often profuse since the lining of the mouth is richly supplied with blood vessels. Blood or bloodstained saliva can be seen hanging from the side of the jaws *(photo 3)*.

Cause
Usually an injury. The dog sometimes bites his tongue during a fight or the mucous membrane, which lines the mouth, may be cut by glass, wire or a piece of bone.

Treatment
Obviously, again a job for your veterinary surgeon. As a first-aid measure the dog should be given a drink of cold water containing a pinch of salt. This will often control the bleeding if the damage is slight.

1
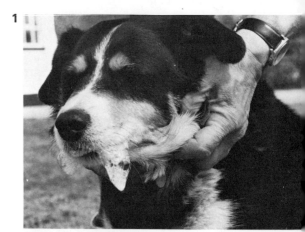

2
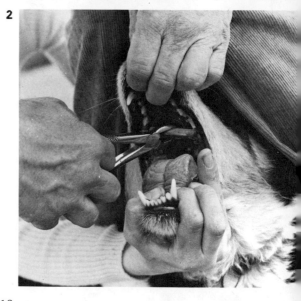

TUMOURS

One of the commonest causes of persistent bleeding is a tumour growth called an epulis, which usually grows out from the gums around the base of a tooth *(photo 4)*.

This will be discovered by the veterinary surgeon during his examination, and he will probably advise surgery.

WARTS

Occasionally in a young adult dog a mass of small white warts, some on a stalk, cover the buccal mucosa (mouth lining). Similar growths can occur in puppies.

Cause

Thought to be a filtrable virus.

Treatment

Very much a matter for your veterinary surgeon although the prognosis (i.e. the outlook) is usually quite good, as the dog's body builds up a powerful natural resistance against the virus which causes the warts. When that resistance reaches a certain level, the warts drop off.

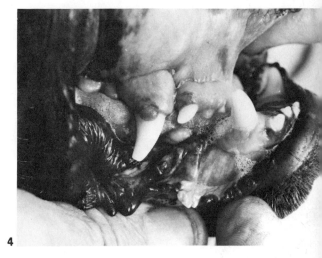

4

ULCERS

Causes

1. Bad teeth.
2. Vitamin B deficiency.
3. Kidney trouble.
4. An infected wound.
5. Leptospirosis (See page 90).

Symptoms

There is usually an offensive smell from the breath *(photo 5)* and the ulcers can be

3

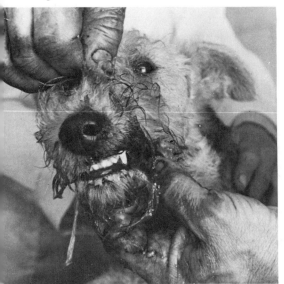

5

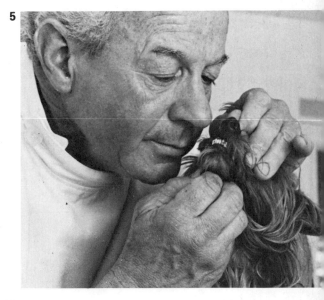

seen chiefly on the upper gums or inside the lips. The dog may slobber and go off his food.

Treatment
Take the patient immediately to a veterinary surgeon, since a correct diagnosis is imperative if the condition is to be cleared up. If the teeth are bad, the patient will be admitted for tooth scaling. If a vitamin deficiency or kidney trouble is suspected, the correct treatment will be prescribed. A wound ulcer may have to be cauterised *(photo 6)*.

BAD BREATH AND NO ULCER

This is common and can be very offensive.

Cause
Where there is no apparent cause, such as tartar and/or ulcers, the condition is usually digestive.

Can it Be Treated?
Yes—very successfully. A week's course of a valuable proprietary drug called Flagyl *(photo 7)*, will clear the condition up for several months. Flagyl is obtained only through a veterinary surgeon.

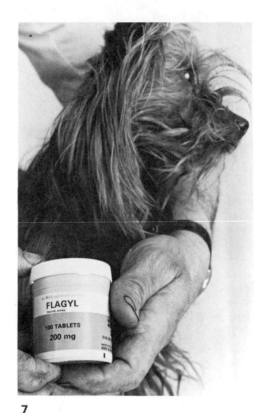

7

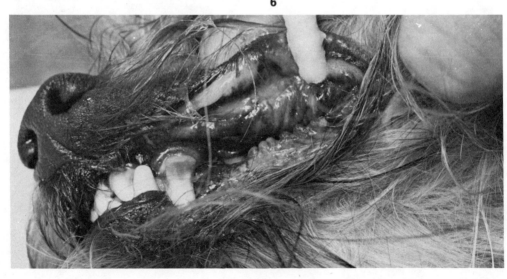

6

31
The Throat

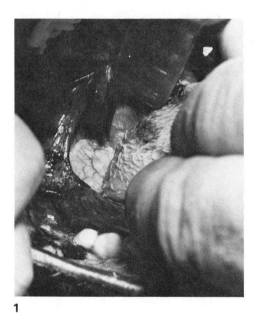

1

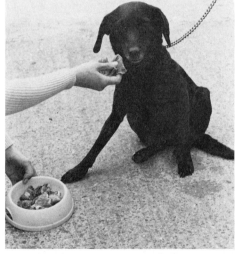

2

TONSILITIS

LIKE HUMANS, dogs have two tonsils one on each side at the back of the throat *(photo 1)*. These tonsils are the first line of defence against any infection entering through the mouth and nose. Tonsilitis occurs when there is an inflammation of one or other or both—usually both.

Cause
Infection by bacteria or viruses.

Symptoms
The first sign is that the dog refuses its food *(photo 2)*—it may or may not cough and has some difficulty in swallowing water.

Usually the temperature is elevated and the patient may salivate or slobber at the mouth.

Veterinary examination reveals the swollen tonsils.

Treatment
A rapid response is usually obtained from a course of antibiotics.

121

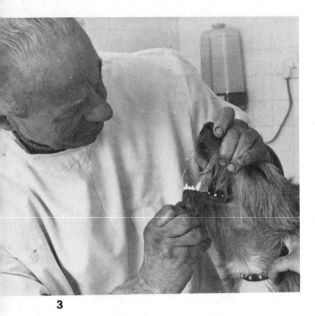

3

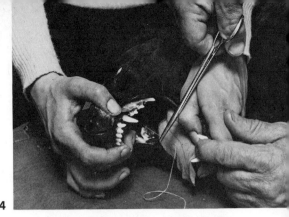

4

PHARYNGITIS

The pharynx is the cavity at the back of the mouth *(photo 3)*. In the dog it is well developed and extremely powerful. Pharyngitis simply means inflammation of this area.

Cause

It is my experience that pharyngitis in the dog occurs chiefly as a result of some injury, e.g. by spicules of bones, stick, glass, needles, etc. or by some corrosive irritant poison.

Symptoms

The patient goes completely off food and salivates profusely. He may even refuse to drink water or milk.

The temperature is usually normal.

A careful examination of the back of the throat will reveal the inflammation; an anaesthetic is usually required to effect such an examination.

Treatment

If a foreign body is present, it is removed *(photo 4)* and antibiotics combined with anti-inflammatory agents are prescribed to control secondary infection.

Forced feeding of water, glucose solution or milk may be necessary for several days till the inflammation subsides sufficiently to allow swallowing; subsequently for a week or so the food should be minced or mashed up.

LARYNGITIS

The larynx or voice box is situated at the back of the throat *(diagram A)*. It controls the entry of air into the trachea,

*Diagram A
The larynx
or throat box.*

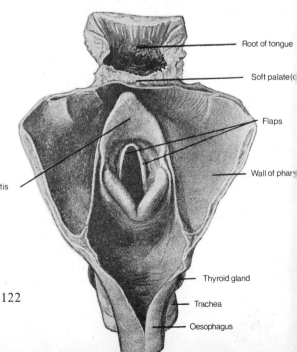

Root of tongue

Soft palate(c

Flaps

Wall of phary

Epiglottis

Thyroid gland

Trachea

Oesophagus

bronchi and lungs and prevents, by means of the epiglottis, food and water from entering therein. Laryngitis occurs when there is an inflammation of this area.

Cause
Bacterial infection secondary to any other debilitating disease. It can occur simultaneously with tonsilitis or tracheitis, but I have rarely diagnosed the condition on its own.

Symptoms
An elevated temperature together with persistent coughing which is exacerbated by pressing on the larynx.

Treatment
A five- or seven-day course of antibiotics will clear the condition spectacularly. Before the days of antibiotics the cure depended entirely on nature and took up to three weeks or longer.

TUMOURS—CANCER

Cancer of the throat, particularly the pharyngeal area *(photo 5)*, is not uncommon in the dog.

Symptoms
Seen mainly in older dogs. The patient goes off food and lies about trembling intermittently. Attempts at drinking water produce attacks of shivering.

When the mouth is forced open the dog

5

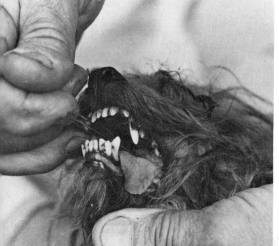

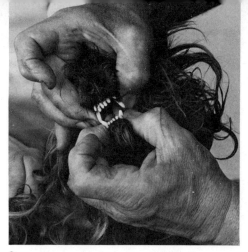

6

howls in anguish *(photo 6)*. However, the diagnosis of this condition requires all the skill of an experienced veterinary surgeon.

Treatment
Euthanasia. Affected dogs are thus much more fortunate than human throat cancer patients.

TRACHEA (WINDPIPE)
The trachea is the length of so-called windpipe which passes from the larynx to the bifurcation of the bronchi *(see diagram B)*. It is lined by a membrane which we

Diagram B.

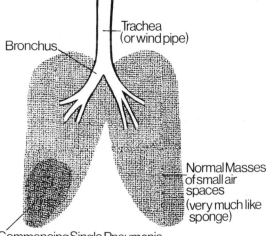

Bronchus

Trachea (or windpipe)

NormalMasses of small air spaces (very much like sponge)

Commencing Single Pneumonia air spaces filled by inflammatory exudate

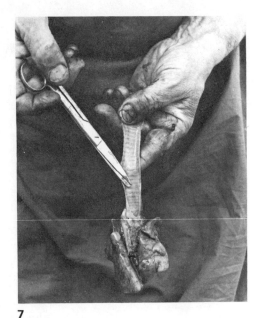

7

call ciliated epithelium *(photo 7)*.

TRACHEITIS
This means inflammation of the tracheal lining. In my experience it is uncommon and extremely difficult to diagnose. This is probably because tracheitis occurs in conjunction with tonsilitis and/or bronchitis.

Cause
Infection by bacteria or direct injury caused by the inhalation of a foreign body.

Symptoms
Persistent coughing for no apparent reason. In a typical tracheitis the dog's temperature is normal.

Treatment
Very much a matter for your veterinary surgeon. Before prescribing anti-inflammatory agents and antibiotics he will probably X-ray the region to eliminate the possibility of a foreign body.

FOREIGN BODY IN TRACHEA AND EPIGLOTTIS
Puppies, particularly, occasionally get a foreign body such as a needle or small spicule of bone lodged in the epiglottis or trachea during the bolting of their food.

Symptoms
The symptoms are violent and continual coughing combined with intermittent rubbing of the throat region with the hind paws. The pup will refuse to eat or drink. Occasionally the blockage closes the air passage completely—the pup chokes and its tongue turns blue.

Treatment
An immediate visit to the veterinary surgeon. If X-ray reveals a foreign body, a general anaesthetic will be required for its removal *(photo 8)*. Fortunately such lodgements usually occur high up within reach of a pair of forceps, though even when low down in the trachea they are accessible by surgery.

8

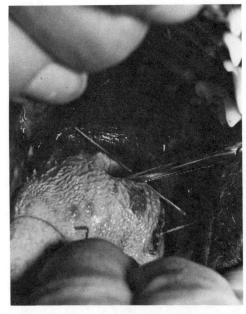

Where the obstruction is complete, the pup's life will depend on how quickly you can get a veterinary surgeon—he will do an emergency tracheotomy, i.e. open up into the windpipe direct to allow air and oxygen into the lungs pending the removal of the object.

Prevention

Never mix small bones with the food of pups and don't leave sewing needles lying about where pups, or for that matter cats, can reach them. Several times I've opened a coughing pup's mouth only to see a tell-tale length of cotton protruding from the back of the throat.

The Bronchi

The bronchi are the two powerful tubes which run from the trachea into the lungs *(see diagram B)*—there they divide and subdivide into masses of ever smaller tubes until eventually they reach the minute air spaces which make the lung so much like a sponge. Like the trachea, the bronchi are lined by ciliated epithelium.

BRONCHITIS

This simply means inflammation of the lining of the bronchi. It is a common condition especially in older dogs, as indeed it is in older human beings.

Cause

Bacterial infection. Bronchitis is a frequent secondary symptom of distemper. (See 'Distemper', page 84).

Symptoms

There are two types: acute and chronic.

In acute bronchitis the dog runs a high fever (105°F/40·5°C or 106°F/41°C), goes off its food and has repeated attacks of violent coughing. It will require a skilled veterinary surgeon to pinpoint the source of the trouble and he will do so by careful auscultation of the chest with his stethoscope.

In chronic bronchitis the temperature is usually normal (101·5°F/38·5°C), and there is a history of repeated attacks. The patient may cough up lumps of sputum; these comprise portions of the damaged broncheal lining.

Treatment

Acute cases usually respond spectacularly to combined antibiotic and anti-inflammatory treatment. In my experience it is wise to blitz such cases in order to prevent recurrence, with the eventual development of the chronic condition which is difficult and unsatisfactory to treat.

Prevention

Since distemper or hard pad infection is one of the commonest causes of bronchitis in the dog, make sure your pup is vaccinated as early as possible and a booster dose of vaccine given at least every two years.

KENNEL COUGH

Recently, in Great Britain, there have been widespread epidemics of coughing in kennels *(photo 9)*. This has been loosely

9

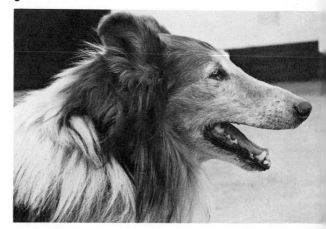

125

designated 'kennel cough' and is in fact a bronchitis with some involvement of the trachea.

Cause
A virus infection, though the virus has not as yet been identified.

Symptoms
Young pups are affected most severely though the trouble can be serious and persistent in older dogs.

There is violent, persistent and often continual coughing. The cough is harsh and dry and can lead to reflex vomiting. For approximately 24 hours there is a rise in temperature to 103°F (39°C) or 104°F (40°C), then it returns to normal and remains so unless a secondary pneumonia flares up.

Treatment
I have found kennel cough difficult and unsatisfactory to treat. Antibiotics by themselves have little or no effect.

From my experience the most important therapy is good feeding and correct housing. At the same time I prescribe cortisone by injection and by the mouth combined with a ten-day antibiotic cover to prevent secondary lung complications. Broad spectrum antibiotics are the most satisfactory.

TUMOURS OF THE BRONCHI
I have never seen a case of bronchial cancer; it would appear that the bronchi are a rare site for tumour growths.

32

Diseases of the Nose and Nasal Passages

RHINITIS *(Inflammation of the Nasal Mucous Membrane)*

THIS CONDITION is also known as nasal catarrh or coryza. It may be acute or chronic.

Cause
Acute catarrh is often an early sign of distemper. It may also flare up on its own due to the inhalation of irritant gases or the invasion of the nostrils by the larvae of certain flies.

The direct cause is the infection of the mucous membrane by organisms. This occurs when the general resistance of the dog or of the membrane is lowered in some way, e.g. by draughts.

Symptoms
Acute
The first sign is usually sneezing. The nostrils run profusely with a clear watery discharge *(photo 1)* which soon changes to a thick white pus.

The inside of the nostrils are swollen and reddened and a conjunctivitis is often present or at least a running eye. This is due to the inflammation closing the lacrimal duct which opens into the nasal cavity.

The temperature is usually up to 103° (39°C) or 103·5°F (39·5°C). (Normal temperature of the dog is 101·5°F/38·5°C).

Chronic
When a discharge from one or both nostrils persists or keeps recurring, the condition is regarded as chronic *(photo 2)*. A foul smell from the pus indicates diseased bone or bad tooth roots. Ulcers may develop on the lining.

Treatment
Take the dog to your veterinary surgeon at once as a correct diagnosis is essential to successful treatment.

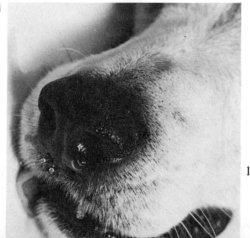

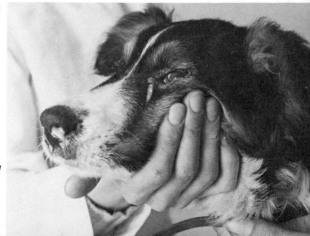

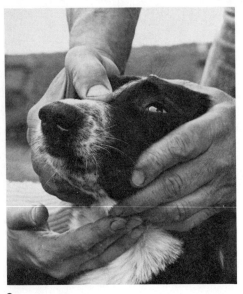

3

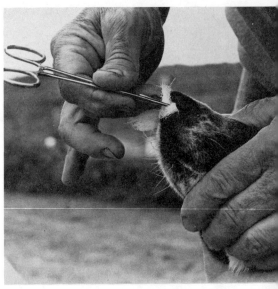

4

As a first-aid measure 'steaming' may be tried. Hold the dog's head over a bowl of hot water to which a teaspoonful of Friar's balsam has been added. Then sponge away all discharge and smear the nostrils with vaseline.

HAEMORRHAGE

Causes

1. Injury producing bleeding from the mucous lining.
2. Persistent sneezing due to inhalation of dust or pepper, etc.
3. Tumour formation in the nasal cavity (usually in older dogs).
4. Violent exercise (e.g. dog racing).

Symptoms

Blood coming from one or both nostrils (*photo 3*). If a tumour is present, the bleeding is usually unilateral and there may be a swelling high up in the nasal cavity.

Treatment

If the haemorrhage is severe consult your veterinary surgeon immediately. Most people do this as the sight of blood usually causes panic.

If slight and coming from one nostril only, the bleeding is only transitory and will probably stop without treatment.

As a first-aid measure, before veterinary treatment, cold water douches may be applied over the bridge of the nose, and if the haemorrhage is severe the nostrils may be plugged with gauze or lint (*photo 4*).

33

The Sinuses

THE SINUSES are cavities found in the skull. These spaces communicate with the nose and their lining is continuous with that of the nasal chambers.

The maxillary sinus is small and directly joined to the nose and is roofed over by the maxilla. The frontal sinus is large in the bigger breeds but comparatively small in the toys. It is roofed by the frontal bone. It has two compartments both of which open into the maxillary sinus *(see diagram)*.

SINUSITIS

Sinusitis means inflammation of the lining of one or both sinuses.

Cause

It may occur when any inflammation of the nasal passages extends into the sinuses or it can be caused by a parasite. Either can lead to a filling up of the sinuses with a bloody discharge or with pus (called empyema). A tumour growth in the sinus can also discharge pus.

Symptoms

Copious or slight but continual purulent discharge from one or both nostrils—usually only from one *(photo 1)*. If the

Diagram A

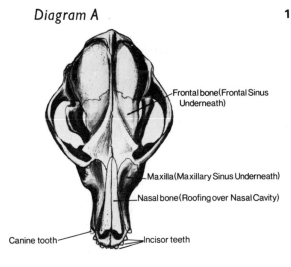

Frontal bone (Frontal Sinus Underneath)

Maxilla (Maxillary Sinus Underneath)

Nasal bone (Roofing over Nasal Cavity)

Canine tooth

Incisor teeth

SKULL OF DOG; DORSAL VIEW.

1

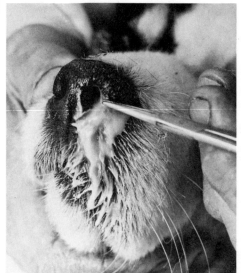

I

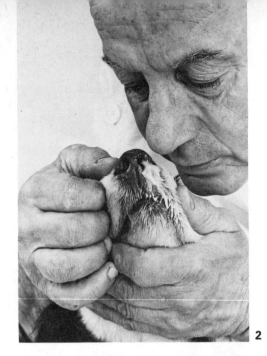

discharge smells badly, then disease of the bone or of a tooth must be suspected *(photo 2)*. The dog may be giddy or hold its head to one side, especially when the frontal sinus is full of pus.

Treatment
Very much a matter for your veterinary surgeon. He may prescribe steaming but will probably have to open directly into the sinuses and drain them from the outside. This will be done under an anaesthetic using an instrument called a trephine *(photo 3)*. If a growth or a parasite is present, they can usually be removed although surgery may not be possible if the growth is malignant.

2

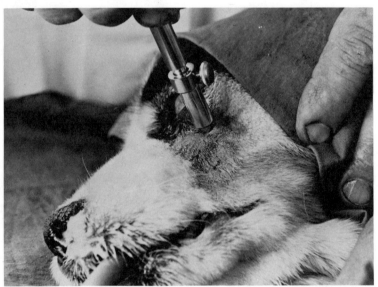

3

34
The Thyroid and Parathyroid Glands

THE THYROID gland is situated in the dog's neck high up and close to the trachea *(photo 1)*.

The thyroid is a ductless gland which secretes a product called thyroxine, which plays a vital part in the nutrition of all parts of the body and especially the hair.

Lying embedded in each thyroid gland or close to it is a pale soft body known as the parathyroid gland. The parathyroids, among other duties, control the calcium blood levels, calcium being one of the two chief minerals on which the work of the muscles depend.

HYPOTHYROIDISM
This means deficiency of thyroxine.

Symptoms
Loss of hair. I have seen dogs completely bald regrowing their entire coat after a daily oral dose of thyroid extract was prescribed (see 'Baldness', page 73).

Thyroid deficiency also causes extreme fatness in old dogs and laziness in bitches towards the end of pregnancy *(photo 2)*.

Treatment
The daily oral (mouth) dosage of tablets containing thyroid extract produce a spectacular recovery but, of course, a skilled veterinary surgeon will be required to diagnose the condition.

Prevention
It is impossible to anticipate thyroid deficiency.

DISTURBANCE OF THE PARATHYROID GLAND
This occurs in eclampsia and in chorea (see 'Canine Distemper', page 84) and epilepsy (see 'Fits', page 197).

In the treatment of each of these conditions it is advantagious to prescribe thyroid and parathyroid extract together with the other drugs recommended.

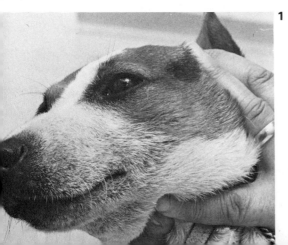

1

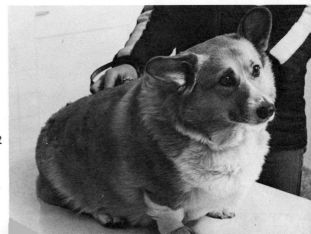

2

35

The Lungs

PNEUMONIA

THE TERM 'pneumonia' simply means a lack of air. As can be seen from the diagram, the lungs are like two sponges—composed of a mass of minute spaces. These fill up with air when the animal breathes in: the oxygen passes from the air into the minute blood vessels which weave an intricate pattern around the thin walls of the tiny air cavities. At the same time, the blood discharges its waste carbon dioxide into the spaces and this is exhaled when the dog breathes out. The oxygen is required for heat, energy and the normal functioning of the entire body: the process is vital and continuous.

Pneumonia occurs when there is damage to the air spaces—damage by injury

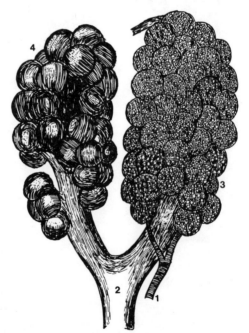

The outer surface of two minute lobules of the lung.

1. Branch of the pulmonary artery ramifying over the air alveoli.
2. The small bronchial tube of the lobule.
3. Capillaries.
4. Air vesicles or alveoli.

132

(traumatic pneumonia) or by inflammation (bacterial pneumonia).

Cause

Traumatic pneumonia is seen as a result of accidents—usually in dogs that have been hit by a car or run over, or shot *(photo 1)*.

Inflammatory pneumonia is due to invasion of the lung tissue by bacteria. This can occur when the dog's resistance is lowered in any way, i.e. by exposure, chills, malnutrition or disease (see 'Distemper').

Another form of pneumonia, where the air spaces fill up with fluid (lymph) occurs in old dogs when the heart becomes incompetent (see 'Cardiac Asthma', page 135); this we call a mechanical pneumonia.

Symptoms

At all times rapid and distressed breathing with or without coughing *(photo 2)*. In bacterial pneumonia the temperature may rise to 106°F (41°C).

Pneumonic breathing is typical—a short intake of air and a longer output usually accompanied by an audible grunt.

Skilled veterinary examination with the stethoscope can detect the areas of lung infected; in the early stages there are unnatural noises (râles) and, later, areas of consolidation.

Treatment

A prolonged course of broad spectrum antibiotics administered and prescribed by your veterinary surgeon as early as possible. The term 'broad spectrum' simply means activity against a wide variety of organisms or bacteria. Such broad spectrum antibiotics are necessary in pneumonias because several really powerful bacteria are usually at work.

Prevention

Canine distemper is the most common predisposing cause of pneumonia in dogs —therefore a rigid vaccination routine should always be adhered to.

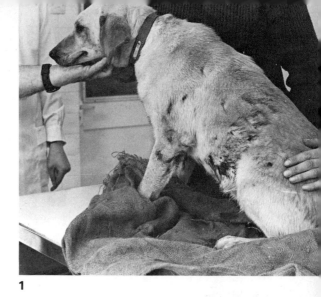

1

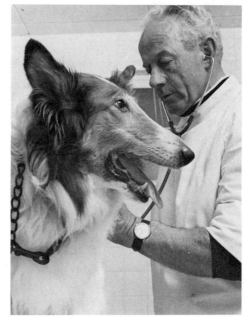

2

CANCER OF THE LUNGS

Cancer of the lungs does occur in dogs but it is not common. In the course of my career I have not seen more than half-a-dozen cases. Probably this is because dogs have enough sense not to smoke! I must admit when I see humans sucking cigarettes and pipes I find myself wondering whether in fact we are, after all, 'higher animals' than dogs.

133

Cause

As always the precise cause of cancer is obscure. Nonetheless it is associated with lowered resistance of the tissues. The few cases I have seen have been in chronic bronchitic or asthmatical ageing dogs.

Symptoms

Similar or virtually identical to a mechanical pneumonia with coughing a constant feature. Usually before the grunting stage is reached, a fairly large part of the lung is involved. Diagnosis is only possible by X-ray done by an experienced veterinary surgeon.

Treatment

Depends entirely on the area involved. If only one lung is affected, then the cancer can be removed together with the whole of that lung. I am pleased to report the apparent success of such an operation on the last case I diagnosed; this patient is still alive nearly two years after the operation.

TUBERCULOSIS

Tuberculosis of the lungs can still occur in dogs, especially in densely populated towns though fortunately, with the decrease in human TB, it is becoming increasingly rare.

Cause

Infection by the tubercle bacillus. At one time the dog frequently picked the bug up from cow's milk, but with this source now closed the bacillus comes from another animal or from a human being.

Symptoms

The symptoms are similar to cancer and asthma, though the persistent coughing is associated with a muco-purulent sputum. The veterinary surgeon diagnoses the condition by examining the sputum microscopically.

Treatment

In dogs, as in humans, tuberculosis can be treated successfully by a prolonged course of streptomycin injections but success depends entirely on an early diagnosis, so if your dog has a chronic cough, and especially if it is coughing up mucus or sputum, get it to a veterinary surgeon immediately. Remember, an infected dog could affect your children.

ASTHMA

There are two types of asthma encountered in dogs—allergic asthma (often inherited, as in humans) and cardiac asthma. It is my experience that of these two, the cardiac type is by far the more common.

ALLERGIC ASTHMA

Cause

A pup is born with an allergy against certain substances usually hairs, dust or pollen.

Symptoms

Repeated attacks of coughing and distressed breathing *(photo 3)*.

3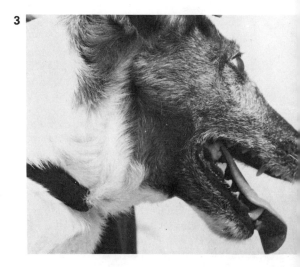

Auscultation of the lungs reveal what we call typical râles, i.e. tinkling, rustling or crackling sounds.

What happens is that the frequent bouts of coughing cause the walls of the minute air spaces to break down until eventually there are large air sacs in the lungs—the air moving in and out of these sacs produce the typical asthmatical lung sounds.

Treatment

Obviously the more frequent the attacks, the more severe they are liable to become and the greater the damage to the lung. I have found that the only drug that controls allergic asthma in dogs is cortisone and it has to be prescribed in very small doses—more or less continuously. Nonetheless it does control it and allows the dog to live out a useful life, comparatively comfortably. Acute attacks can be controlled by injecting long-acting cortisone.

CARDIAC ASTHMA

Cause

This condition, seen almost entirely in old dogs, is due to the heart not functioning properly. Since the blood is not passing round the body as quickly as it should, the waste products that normally filter through into the lymphatics or drainage vessels (the lymphatics run alongside the veins) seep out into the surrounding tissues. When this happens lymphatic or dropsical fluid fills up the air spaces in the lungs, producing in reality a mechanical pneumonia.

Symptoms

The first sign invariably reported by the owners is coughing. There is usually a history of age and the dog apparently tiring 'more quickly than it used to'.

Examination of the lungs and heart by an experienced veterinary surgeon reveals the cardiac fault and the fluid splashings in the lungs usually towards the lung base *(photo 4)*.

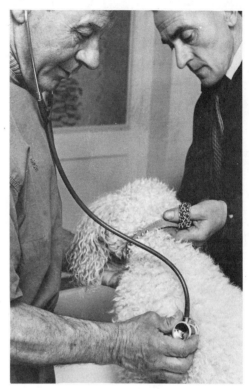

4

In advanced cases the patient is in great distress and may be unable to lie down for more than a few seconds. Dropsical fluid can be detected in the abdomen and underneath the skin.

Prognosis

If treatment is started early enough, the patient can be kept going happily for several years. In fact recently I put a 17-year-old dog to sleep which I had been treating successfully for six years.

Treatment

This has to be continuous and done only under the supervision of your veterinary surgeon.

Heart stimulants plus diuretics comprise the basis of all successful treatment.

The heart drugs speed up the circulation and the diuretics increase the fluid loss through the kidneys. But, as I say above, the treatment has to be continuous with a daily dosing routine, though once progress is established it means merely the owner calling at monthly intervals to report to the veterinary surgeon and collect a fresh supply of tablets.

Acute cases can be relieved by injecting the diuretic, especially where abdominal dropsy is present *(photo 5)*.

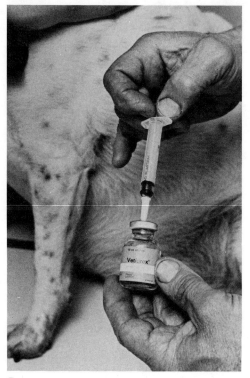

5

36
Unusual Chest Conditions

THERE ARE several of these but the only reasonably common one and certainly the only one likely to be encountered in the adult dog is:

DIAPHRAGMATIC HERNIA
This occurs when the powerful muscular diaphragm which separates the chest from the abdominal cavity becomes torn or divided in any way *(photo 1)*.

Cause
Almost invariably a car accident, though I have seen a diaphragmatic hernia resulting from a dog stretching itself during the jumping of a high fence *(photo 2)*.

Symptoms
Not unlike those seen in asthma—intermittent bouts of coughing and respiratory distress, particularly after a walk or run around. The dog may have difficulty in settling comfortably anywhere.

The veterinary surgeon will hear abnormal noises in the chest and will X-ray after feeding a barium meal.

Treatment
Immediate surgery provides a very real chance of complete recovery. Certainly undue delay can cause death. If the dog attempts to walk or run down a slope, the entire abdominal contents may slip into the chest and cause death by pressure suffocation.

The operation is a major one. It can be tackled through the abdomen or through the chest, but either way the tear in the diaphragm is extremely difficult to get to and even more difficult to repair.

General Advice
If after a road accident, your dog suffers respiratory distress or bouts of coughing, take it to a veterinary surgeon immediately.

2

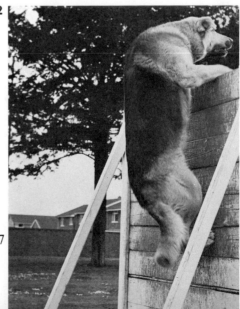

1

37
The Heart and Blood Vessels

THE BEAT of a dog's heart is irregular and it requires a great deal of experience to recognise normality. Obviously, therefore, the diagnosis of heart conditions has to be left to the veterinary surgeon. There are, however, a number of simple cardiac symptoms which an observant owner can spot and probably save his pet's life by doing so.

We have already dealt with probably the most common, viz. those of cardiac asthma, but there are at least two other syndromes to watch out for, especially in ageing working dogs or at any time after a prolonged debilitating disease.

VALVULAR DISEASE

The circulation of the dog's blood is identical to that seen in man and in all other classes of animals.

The deoxygenated blood is carried by the veins from every part of the body and passes through two large veins—the an-

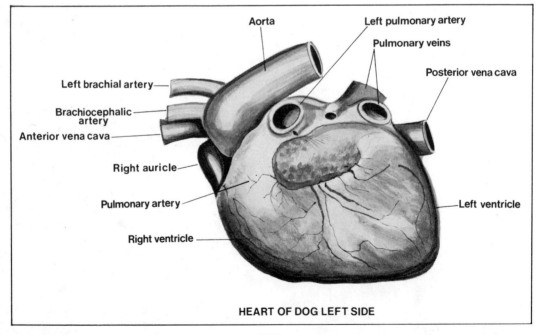

HEART OF DOG LEFT SIDE

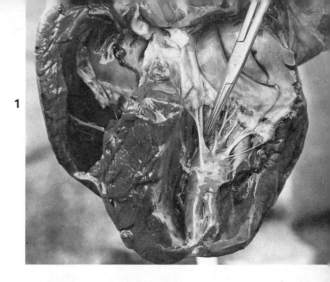

terior and posterior venae cavae *(see diagram)* into the right auricle of the heart.

From the right auricle the blood, still without oxygen is passed (by contraction of the right auricle wall) through what is called the bicuspid valve into the right ventricle.

From the right ventricle the blood is pumped (by contraction of the right ventricular wall) through the pulmonary artery (which divides into two) to the lungs. There, in the minute air sacs of the lungs, the blood gives off its waste carbon dioxide and takes up its supply of oxygen.

It then passes back through five or six pulmonary veins, to the left auricle of the heart.

From there it is pumped through the tricuspid valve into the left ventricle *(photo 1)*.

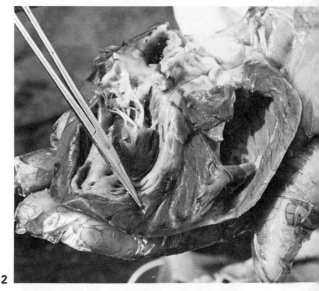

When the left ventricle contracts the blood is pumped through the aorta (the largest of the body's arteries) to every part of the body.

The process is continuous throughout the whole of the dog's life. Obviously, since the ventricles have to do most of the work, their walls are much thicker than those of the auricles with the left ventricular wall a massive powerful structure *(photo 2)*.

In addition to the bicuspid and tricuspid valves, valves are present at the entry and exit of all the heart veins and arteries.

Valvular disease occurs when any one of these hard working valves becomes incompetant.

CONGENITAL VALVULAR DISEASE

Pups are sometimes born with an incompetant bicuspid or tricuspid valve.

Symptoms

Inertia *(photo 3)*—they sleep a lot, tire rapidly, breathe heavily after even mild exercise and their tongue and mucous

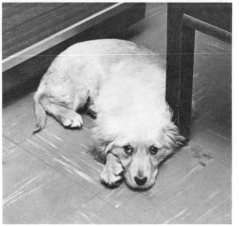

139

membranes (linings of the mouth, nostrils and eyes) turn blue.

This is exactly the same syndrome as the 'blue-baby' in humans.

Treatment
Surgical insertion of a plastic valve in place of the incompetant one. So far this is exotic surgery done experimentally only, but I anticipate in the future many small animal surgeons in this country and throughout the world performing this operation as regularly and successfully as the human surgeons.

Heart stimulants *(photo 4)* have little beneficial effect.

VALVULAR DISEASE IN ADULT DOGS
This is most likely to occur in working dogs that have led a strenuous hard life, though I have often seen it develop in comparatively sedentary lap dogs.

Symptoms
The symptoms are identical to those des-cribed with the following important addi-tion. When the adults get valvular in-competance the heart bulges out inter-mittently (cardiac hypertension). This pro-duces a sharp pain which causes the dog to howl out for no apparent reason—a pain identical to that occurring in so-called angina pectoris in humans.

Sometimes the dog will 'flake out' for varying periods during the attack.

Treatment
Very much a matter for your veterinary surgeon. In ageing adults the condition can be alleviated by drugs designed to slow down the circulation but their appli-cation requires considerable skill in diag-nosis plus knowledge and experience.

CORONARY THROMBOSIS
This is a thrombus or blood clot which forms in one of the main heart vessels *(photo 5)*.

This does occur in dogs but not nearly so often as it does in humans, probably

4

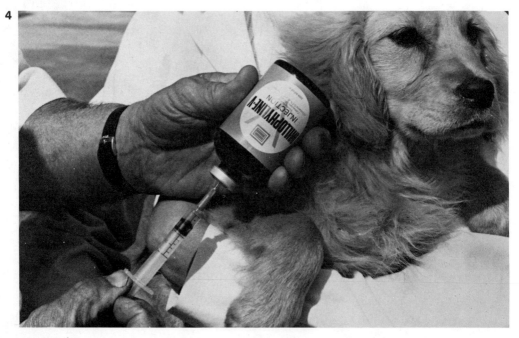

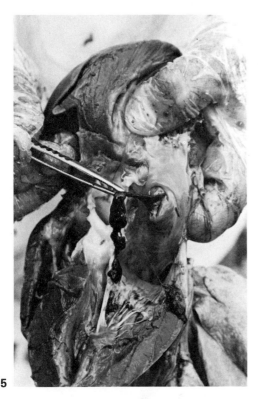

5

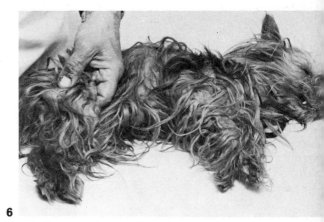

6

because the average dog is more sensibly fed and gets more exercise than the average man or woman.

Symptoms
To the lay person these are indistinguishable from those described for valvular incompetance, though the blueness of the membranes is rarely seen.

A sharp cry out followed by an apparent fainting fit are the signs to look out for *(photo 6)*. If the thrombus is complete the dog is soon dead.

Treatment
If it recovers from the attack, get it to a veterinary surgeon as soon as possible.

He will diagnose thrombosis if he can detect no valvular trouble.

The treatment is identical to that used in humans—drugs to slow the circulation down plus drugs to prevent the blood clotting.

Heart Transplants in Dogs?
These are by no means an impossibility for the future. Much of the experimental transplant surgery has been carried out in dogs.

Obviously, at the moment such general surgery would be an economic nightmare.

38
The Stomach

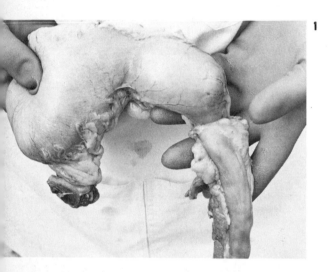

1 THE STOMACH of the dog is a well-developed organ *(photo 1)* suited to coping with carnivorous foods and with a capacity of 2½ to 5 pints, depending on the breed. As in man and all other animals, the stomach is lined with what we call mucous membrane, but unlike most the dog's mucous membrane is wholly glandular, i.e. every part of it secretes digestive juices *(photo 2)*. Probably because of this the dog tends to vomit more easily than any other class of animal, except perhaps the cat whose stomach has a similar structure.

GASTRITIS

This occurs when there is an inflammation of the highly glandular mucous membrane *(photo 3)*.

2

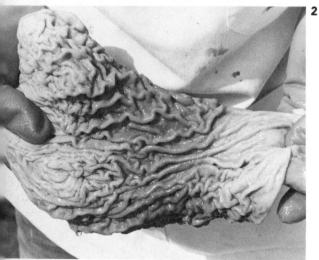

3

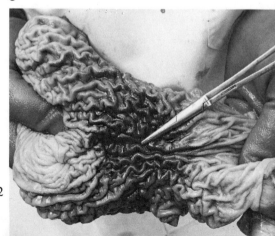

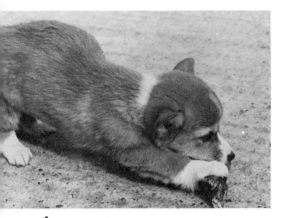

4

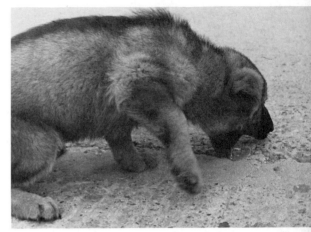

5

Cause

Because of the instinctive habit of foraging, young pups particularly tend to eat rubbish of all kinds *(photo 4)*; inevitably this produces a gastritis.

The more serious types are caused by bacteria, and here again the source is most likely to be old bones or putrefying flesh. The bacteria involved here are both powerful and difficult to control, viz. the salmonella and the *Clostridium botulinum*.

Viruses are also involved; in fact, in recent years, most cases I have had to deal with have been due to virus infection apparently of the contagious type.

Symptoms

Vomiting is the classic sign, though an odd case of vomiting can be disregarded because a normal dog often vomits spontaneously for no apparent reason.

In gastritis the vomiting is violent and persistent *(photo 5)*; the dog is completely off food but will usually constantly seek water, only to vomit it back immediately.

The tongue, particularly the front portion, turns a brown colour and the animal becomes depressed and dehydrated.

The temperature is normal or subnormal except in canine distemper (see 'Distemper', page 84).

Where bacteria and viruses are involved, an enteritis is often present simultaneously (see 'Enteritis', page 147).

Treatment

An immediate visit to your veterinary surgeon; nothing can be more distressing than persistent vomiting.

The veterinary surgeon will inject an antispasmodic or heavy dose of tranquilliser *(photo 6)* which will stop the vomiting more or less immediately. He will then follow that up with drugs by the mouth to control and destroy any bacterial infection.

During treatment there should be no

6

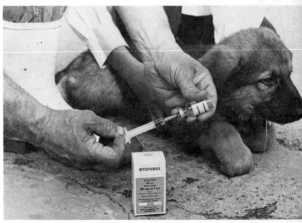

access to solid food for at least 24 hours, though sugar and water or milk should be available ad lib to counteract the dehydration.

In average cases the dog can be returned to solid food on the second day but in rationed quantities. I usually advise three small feeds a day of easily digested protein—eggs or meat (raw if the dog will take it); after a further 48 hours the patient can go back to normal feeding.

Prevention
Since one of the most persistent types of gastritis is that occurring in distemper—NEVER fail to keep your dog fully protected.

*   *   *

Two questions I am repeatedly asked by clients are:

Why do puppies eat everything and anything and, more particularly, why do they eat their own motions (photo 7)?

It is instinctive for all pups to chew at everything—such instinct is borne of a combination of curiosity and a need to develop the jaws and teeth. If, however, they actually swallow the rubbish, then they are hungry—probably short of protein. Such pups are usually fed on biscuits,

meal or cereals with an extremely limited quantity of protein. The simple cure is to feed a correct protein diet (see 'Feeding', page 15).

The eating of motions, however, presents a different problem. This is the condition known as coprophagy and is due to a deficiency of vitamin B. The cure?—yeast tablets given twice daily, raw green vegetables mixed in with each feed and 2 oz (56 g) of raw liver at least twice a week.

In many cases of coprophagy I have seen also a deficiency of the mineral phosphorus. This can be rectified by the addition of the daily diet of two teaspoonsful of sterilised bone flour.

The chief source of phosphorus in the dog's diet is bones and this provides one more reason why the adolescent dog particularly should be allowed to chew at one large bone per week.

FOREIGN BODIES IN THE STOMACH

Cause
Many pups and even adults, particularly of the retrieving breeds, continually chase after stones and sticks thrown by their

7

8

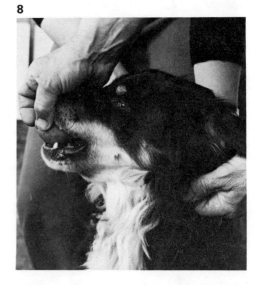

child companions *(photo 8)*. It is a time-honoured game enjoyed by both. Unfortunately sooner or later many of the stones are swallowed and pass into the stomach.

Young dogs often swallow a variety of objects—buttons, coins, small table-tennis balls, lumps of rubber balls, golf balls, etc.

Symptoms

If the foreign body is not sharp edged, it can remain in the stomach for a long time without producing any symptoms at all. Practically all stomach foreign body cases I have seen have been brought to my notice only because the owner actually saw the object disappearing.

Diagnostic symptoms only appear when the foreign body gets lodged in the intestine (See 'Foreign Body in Intestines', page 183).

Treatment

Confirmation of the situation of the object by X-ray followed by the injection of an emetic to make the dog vomit *(photo 9)*. If the patient will eat, I prescribe a heavy meal an hour before I inject the emetic, and in the vast majority of cases I have succeeded in recovering the foreign body.

If sharp edges or pointed—a needle or piece of glass—an immediate operation is indicated.

The operation is called gastrotomy and comprises merely opening up the stomach. Done under a general anaesthetic it is spectacularly successful.

STOMACH TUMOURS

Cancer of the stomach is rare in dogs. I personally have seen only one case and that was part of a widespread infection.

Symptoms

The symptoms would be those of a chronic gastritis.

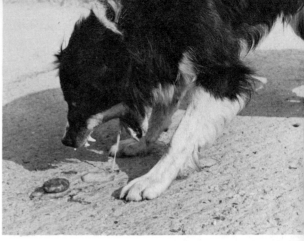

9

Diagnosis
Could be made only by barium X-ray.

Treatment
Left entirely to the discretionary advice of the veterinary surgeon.

PYLORIC CONSTRICTION

As can be seen from the diagram, the pylorus of the stomach is that part where it joins the duodenum. Occasionally pups are born with a pylorus which does not function.

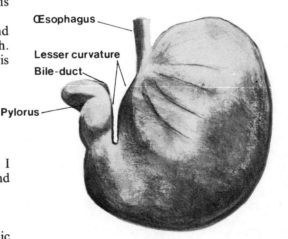

Œsophagus

Lesser curvature

Bile-duct

Pylorus

STOMACH OF A DOG

Symptoms

Persistent vomiting despite any form of treatment. The pup will not thrive or grow and will rapidly become dejected and dehydrated.

Treatment

Whenever you have a pup showing these symptoms, get it to a veterinary surgeon immediately.

A comparatively simple operation comprising controlled cutting through the pyloric muscles will produce a complete cure.

There are two other congenital defects in pups which produce identical symptoms, viz. a persistent aortic arch and an abnormal oesophagus, but both these are uncommon and in any case can only be diagnosed by a veterinary surgeon using X-rays *(photo 10)* or surgery.

Obviously, therefore, if your pup is persistently vomiting he or she should be placed under veterinary supervision as soon as possible.

DILATATION AND TORSION OF THE STOMACH

This may occur in dogs of any breed but by far the greatest incidence is in large deep chested animals *(photo 11)*.

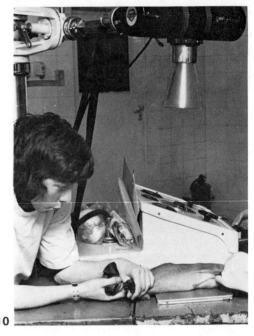

10

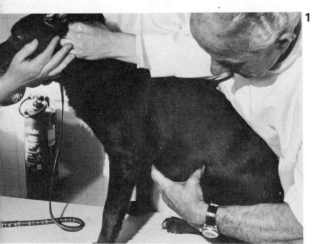

11

Cause

The cause is obscure. The condition may flare up at any time but usually occurs within 6 hours of eating and appears most often in dogs fed once daily.

What Happens?

The stomach fills up rapidly with gases and fluid and twists on itself.

Symptoms

Desperate attempts at vomiting, progressive swelling up of the (in advanced cases) abdomen and distressed breathing; the tongue and mucous membranes of the mouth become cyanosed (purple) and the dog collapses.

Treatment

This is a real emergency; send for your veterinary surgeon immediately. He will probably pass a stomach tube to relieve the distension and operate at once.

Prevention

Although there is no certain preventative, twice daily feeding is the logical and sensible approach.

39
The Intestines

THE INTESTINES of the dog comprise a duodenum, jejunum and ileum (small intestines) and caecum, colon, rectum and anus (large intestines) *(photo 1)*. They are comparatively short.

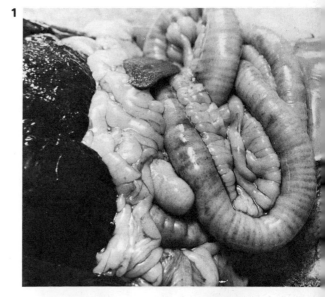

The function of the small intestine is the digestion and absorption of the foodstuffs. In common with all meat-eating animals, the dog has a tough digestive tract and intestinal troubles are rare.

The most common one ('Foreign Body') is dealt with on page 183.

ENTERITIS
This simply means inflammation of the bowel lining. There are two types—acute and chronic.

Cause
Invasion of the mucous membrane by bacteria or damage caused by an irritant poison (see 'Arsenical Poisoning').

Symptoms
Acute diarrhoea *(photo 2)* and abdominal pain. Vomiting is usually present since the stomach is nearly always involved (gastroenteritis). When blood is present in the vomit or faeces (dung) the condition is known as 'haemorrhagic'.

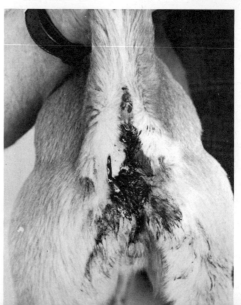

147

Treatment
Injections of tranquillisers combined with broad spectrum antibiotics followed by the oral administration of antibiotics and kaolin.

CHRONIC ENTERITIS
Seen mainly in pups up to the age of 10 months *(photo 3)*.

Cause
The chief cause in my experience is a heavy roundworm infestation.

Symptoms
Persistent sloppy motion and loss in condition.

Treatment
Two doses of roundworm medicine *(photo 4)* at a ten day interval combined with kaolin or charcoal mixed with the food.

It is always best to consult your veterinary surgeon, however, since a tapeworm may be present.

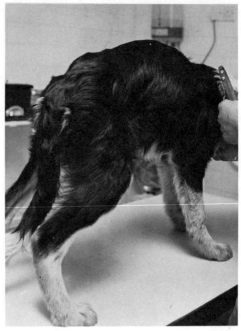

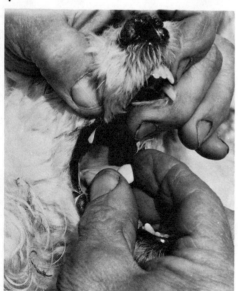

COLITIS
This is another type of chronic enteritis seen in dogs of any age.

Cause
Inflammation of the lining of the colon (part of the large intestine). It may occur secondary to a debilitating disease.

Symptoms
Persistent sloppy motions containing a clear jelly-like substance *(photo 5)*. This clear jelly is part of the mucous lining of the colon.

Treatment
Careful dieting plus a three-month course of charcoal powder given with each meal. I advise three protein meals a day—eggs, meat, chicken or cheese, together with a minute quantity of raw green vegetable, each laced with a level teaspoonful of powdered charcoal.

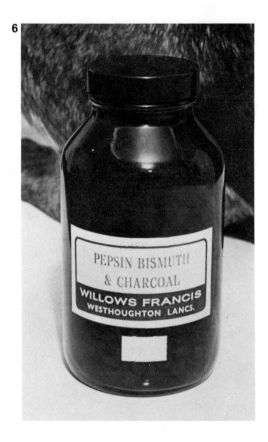

6

A compound digestive tablet containing pepsin and bismuth as well as charcoal provides an ideal substitute for the powdered charcoal on its own *(photo 6)*.

INTUSSUSCEPTION

This is without doubt the most painful of all intestinal obstructions; fortunately it occurs almost exclusively in pups.

In intussusception a portion of the intestine enters within that part immediately above or below itself, i.e. the bowel telescopes on itself.

Cause

In puppies appears to be a heavy roundworm infestation and/or diarrhoea, though it often occurs spontaneously for no apparent reason.

Symptoms

Acute pain and rapid death if not treated quickly. The pup contorts itself with pain and the abdomen swells up *(photo 7)*.

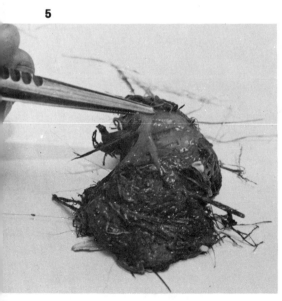

5

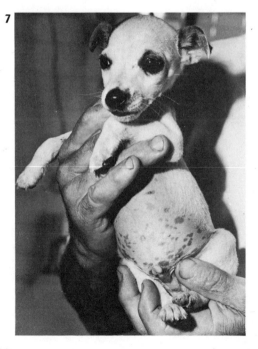

7

Treatment

An emergency trip to a veterinary surgeon. He will identify the telescoped bowel by palpation of the abdomen (probing it with his fingers—*photo 9*) and will operate immediately.

Operation comprises opening into the abdomen under a general anaesthetic and removing the entire telescoped portion.

Prevention

Regular routine worming and feeding. (See 'Worming', page 80, and 'Feeding', page 15).

PROLAPSED ANUS

Seen mostly in pups.

Cause

Persistent diarrhoea and/or heavy round-worm infestatiion; very occasionally, constipation.

Symptoms

The inside lining of the anus and probably the lower part of the rectum protrude from the anus like an angry strawberry. The pup may be in considerable distress and lick the protrusion incessantly.

Treatment

The veterinary surgeon will replace the prolapse and suture it in position.

I always use local anaesthetic for this job and suture with a double anal purse-string suture leaving a thermometer in the rectum to guide me as to what opening is being left.

I then provide a seven-day cover of antibiotic by injection to control infection. I find this latter precaution vital to the success of the operation.

CANCER OF THE INTESTINAL TRACT

The only other intestinal condition of note is cancer and the most common site of intestinal cancer in the dog is the rectum.

Symptoms

Seen almost exclusively in older dogs.

The first sign is usually constipation.

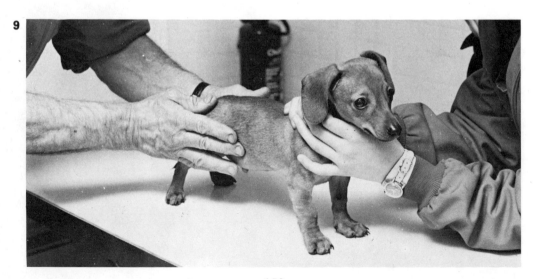

The dog will repeatedly strain to pass a motion just as though he had a mass of bone stuck and he will often squeal out with pain when he does so.

Diagnosis is made by a rectal examination done by the veterinary surgeon *(photo 10)*.

Treatment
Like most internal cancers in the dog, rectal cancer is inoperable but it is also intensely painful and requires immediate euthanasia.

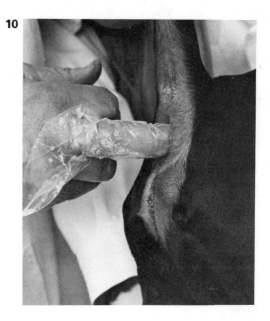

10

40
Bowel and Anal Disorders

PROSTATITIS

THERE IS one other common bowel obstruction seen mainly in old dogs and of course only in *male* dogs (never in bitches) and that is due to an inflammation and enlargement of the prostate gland.

The prostate gland is an accessory sexual gland seen only in males.

Symptoms

The dog, usually a middle-aged or older one, has difficulty in passing motions. He squats for prolonged periods without success *(photo 1)*. He is uncomfortable and often goes off his food and tends to vomit.

Treatment

Immediate veterinary attention is required.

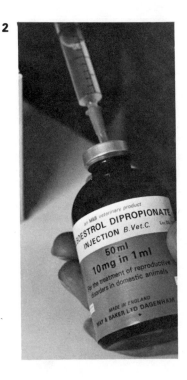

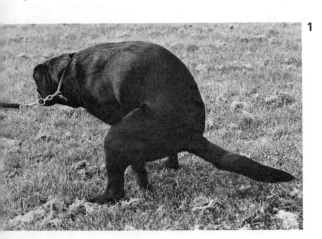

The veterinary surgeon will confirm the diagnosis by rectal examination and will inject and prescribe large doses of female hormone *(photo 2)*.

The enlargement of the prostate in the male is often due to cancerous growth apparently triggered off and exacerbated by ageing male hormones. Large doses of female hormones reverses the process

in the vast majority of cases, though the
the condition does tend to recur.

To avoid this, and often as a routine
therapy, the veterinary surgeon will advise
castration.

BONES STUCK IN RECTUM

The final common intestinal obstruction
is when masses of partially chewed bones
block up the lower part of the rectum.

Symptoms

These are identical to those seen in
prostatitis but the patient is usually
younger. Rectal examination reveals the
impacted bones; often blood denotes
damage to the mucous membrane *(photo
3)*.

Treatment

Very much a matter for your veterinary
surgeon. He will prescribe liquid paraffin
by the mouth and will probably hospitalise

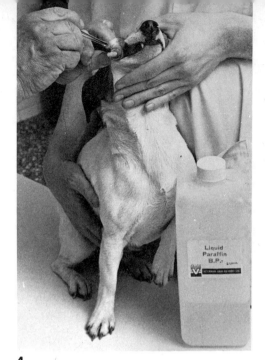

4

the dog for as long as it takes to clear the
rectum *(photo 4)*.

Personally I use repeated liquid paraffin
enemas.

The liquid paraffin has a soothing
lubricating effect.

In bad cases I use whelping forceps, or
the handle of a teaspoon in conjunction
with the liquid paraffin enema, to break
down the impaction and ease it portion by
portion through the anus.

A great deal of experience and patience
is required to avoid permanent damage to
the rectum and anus; as I say, it is very
much a job for a veterinary surgeon.

3

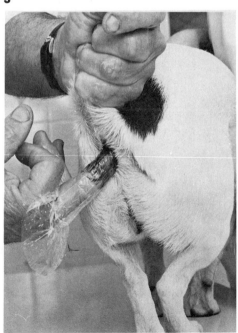

IMPACTION OF THE
ANAL GLANDS

This is without doubt the commonest
condition we have to deal with in canine
practice.

Symptoms

The first sign is usually the dog dragging
his hind quarters along the floor or carpet.
He may be lying quiet then suddenly

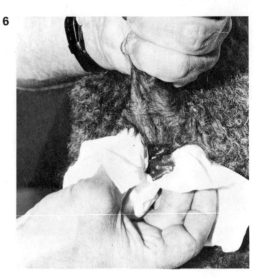

6

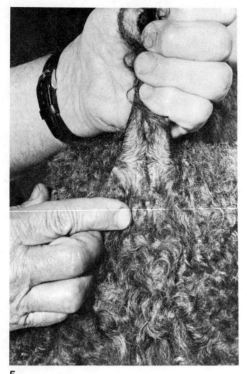

5

squeal out and rush forward to another part of the room.

A persistent Old Wives' Tale has it that such symptoms are caused by worms and often the owner mentions worms when such cases are presented to us.

Cause

On either side of the dog's anus is a gland called the anal gland *(photo 5)*. These glands secrete a foul-smelling lubricating fluid obviously intended to be emptied into the anus each time the dog passes a motion.

Because of present-day feeding most dogs have outlived the use of these glands —the motion is too soft to require them. The result is they fill up and become impacted.

Treatment

Take the patient to a veterinary surgeon

immediately. He will express the foul-smelling contents *(photo 6)* and will inject antibiotics or iodine solution into the glands.

If the condition persists and causes the dog continual trouble, the veterinary surgeon may remove the glands surgically.

My best results have been obtained by injecting a solution of Lugol's iodine into the glands after expressing once a week for three weeks. This appears to destroy the secreting cells which line the glands and to stop the secretion of the contents *(photo 7)*.

7

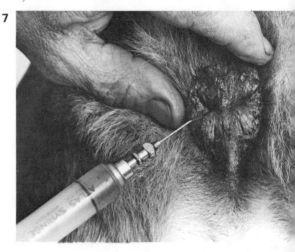

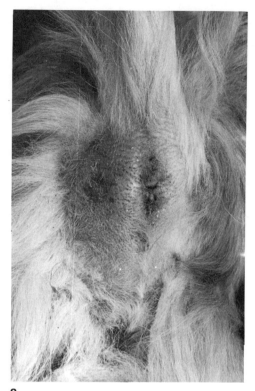

8

ABSCESS AT THE ANUS

Not infrequently an anal gland becomes infected; when this happens an abscess forms.

Symptoms
The dog shows signs of acute pain, especially when attempting to pass a motion. He will squeal or bite when his tail or hind end is handled.

Examination shows a large painful swelling on one side of the anus *(photo 8)*. The dog's temperature is often elevated to around 105°F (40·5°C) or 106°F (41°C) (normal 101·5°F/38·5°C).

Treatment
Because of the inflammation it is not possible to empty the gland by expressing in the usual way, so the abscess has to be

lanced. Obviously this is a job for the veterinary surgeon.

Prevention
Impaction and anal abscesses can be prevented by three-monthly visits to your veterinary surgeon for routine examination and expression of the anal glands.

ANAL FISSURE

One condition that can be mistaken for an early stage anal abscess is a fissure of the anal ring.

Cause
The fissure is an infected ulcerating wound and the original wound has most likely been caused by the passing of sharp pieces of bone.

Symptoms
Identical to those seen in an anal abscess with, in addition, howls of acute agony when the dog squats to pass a motion.

Treatment
In my experience, surgery is the only complete answer to this condition. The ulcerating infected area is completely removed. Repeated caustic dressings may be tried and are occasionally successful *(photo 9)*.

9

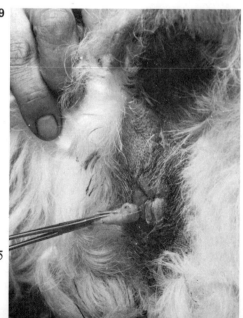

HAEMORRHOIDS

A haemorrhoid or pile is a varicose vein in the rectum, and when this occurs, the symptoms of pain and distress at the hind end can be identical to those seen with an anal abscess or a fissure. However, it is seen mainly in old fat dogs and is never quite so serious as in humans.

Cause

In my experience, the cause is due to repeated attacks of constipation due to the persistent chewing of bones.

Diagnosis and Treatment

These must be left to a skilled veterinary surgeon.

Prevention

The condition can be avoided by rationing the dog to one large thigh bone a week. The dog will enjoy chewing the large bone; this will keep his teeth healthy but he will be unlikely to swallow enough of the bone to produce constipation.

ANAL ADENOMA

An anal adenoma is a small tumour which appears at the anus, usually under the tail, in both dogs and bitches—usually when the animals are ageing *(photo 10)*.

Symptoms

The patient will be seen to be licking at the rear end and examination will reveal the tumour.

Treatment

This type of tumour like that occurring in the prostate gland often responds to treatment by moderate doses of female hormone—weekly injections for three or four weeks plus oral doses.

Personally I prefer to remove the tumour, though I do use hormones sometimes to reduce the growth to operable size.

Repeated injections of female hormones appear to trigger off kidney inflammation.

A comparatively new technique called cryo surgery, which comprises the 'freezing of the growth with nitrous oxide may well prove the complete answer to the problem. *(photo 11)*. The cryo surgery may have to be repeated in three weeks.

10

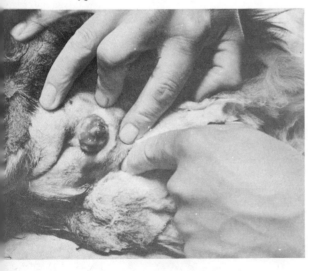

11

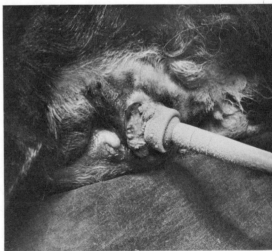

41
The Liver

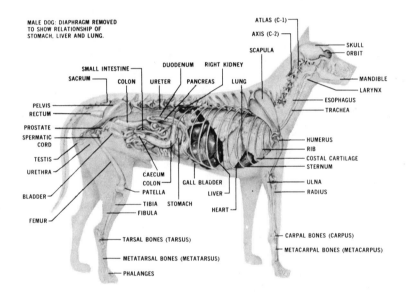

MALE DOG: DIAPHRAGM REMOVED
TO SHOW RELATIONSHIP OF
STOMACH, LIVER AND LUNG.

ATLAS (C-1)
AXIS (C-2)
SCAPULA
SKULL
ORBIT
SMALL INTESTINE
DUODENUM RIGHT KIDNEY
MANDIBLE
LARYNX
SACRUM
COLON URETER PANCREAS LUNG
ESOPHAGUS
TRACHEA
PELVIS
RECTUM
PROSTATE
SPERMATIC
CORD
HUMERUS
RIB
COSTAL CARTILAGE
STERNUM
TESTIS
URETHRA
CAECUM
COLON
GALL BLADDER
ULNA
RADIUS
BLADDER
PATELLA
LIVER
TIBIA STOMACH
FIBULA
HEART
FEMUR
CARPAL BONES (CARPUS)
TARSAL BONES (TARSUS)
METACARPAL BONES (METACARPUS)
METATARSAL BONES (METATARSUS)
PHALANGES

THE LIVER could be described as the factory of the body *(see above)*. It is here that the basic foodstuffs—simple proteins, carbohydrates, minerals and vitamins—are brought to for elaboration and build up before being conveyed to the specific needs of different parts of the body. It vies with the heart, therefore, in importance and work-rate.

Considering the vast amount of work it does and the tremendous importance of its role, liver disease is rare. The two infectious diseases which play havoc with the liver cells, leptospirosis and virus hepatitis, are dealt with fully in another part of this book, but apart from these I can honestly say that I encounter a liver problem in a dog only very occasionally.

Such rare conditions have been, in order of occurrence—cancer, liver abscess and tuberculosis.

CANCER OF THE LIVER
Symptoms
Marked depression, vomiting and completely off food.

157

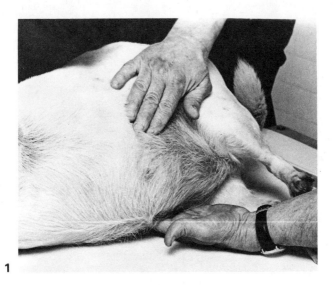

1

The membranes of the mouth and eye are pallid and tinged with yellow.

Ascites can usually be detected. Ascites means abdominal dropsy *(photo 1)*— lymph that has accumulated in the belly cavity simply because of the obstruction produced by cancer of the lymphatic glands which serve the liver.

2

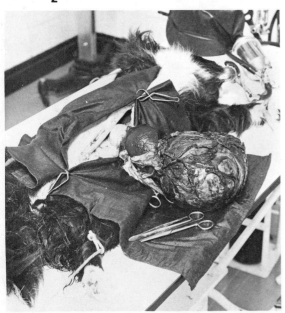

Careful examination of the abdomen by a veterinary surgeon reveals the enlarged and hardened liver and the diagnosis is confirmed by X-ray.

Treatment

Liver cancers are not always hopeless. I advise an immediate exploratory laparotomy, i.e. opening the abdomen to see the extent of the growth *(photo 2)*.

If a reasonable amount of normal liver tissue remains, I do not hesitate to remove the diseased portion. A number of such cases have survived happily for several years after the operation.

LIVER ABSCESS

Cause

A liver abscess can develop secondary to any infection or it can flare up as a result of the migration of parasitic larvae (see 'Internal Parasitic Diseases', page 79).

Symptoms

These only appear when the abscess assumes a size big enough to interfere with the liver's work ratio.

The symptoms are then identical to those seen in cancer.

Treatment
Exploratory laparotomy and removal of diseased tissues; although I have operated only on a few such cases, the percentage success rate has been high.

TUBERCULOSIS
Many years ago, in the 1930s, when a student working in Glasgow clinics, I saw three or four cases a week of liver TB in dogs. In recent years the condition has become a rarity.

Symptoms
Identical to those described for cancer.

Treatment
Exploratory laparotomy followed by euthanasia. In liver TB the entire substance is dotted over with diseased foci.

42

The Spleen

THE SPLEEN is a highly vascular organ situated close to the stomach *(photo 1)*. It has no duct leading from it and its function is not clearly understood.

It appears to play a part in manufacturing red and white blood corpuscles and in destroying the old worn out red corpuscles. However, its functions are not vital to the body since the entire spleen can be removed without endangering the animal's life.

The two splenic problems that arise in dog practice are:
1. Rupture of the Spleen.
2. Splenic Tumour.

RUPTURE OF THE SPLEEN

This is frequently seen in road accident cases *(photo 2)*.

1

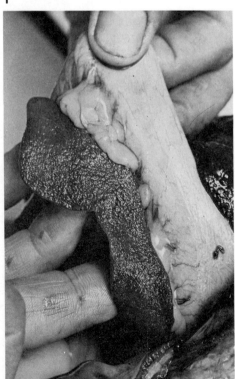

2

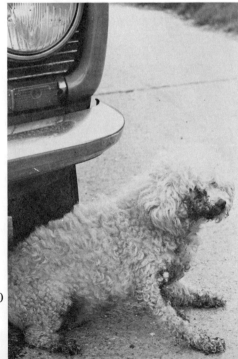

Symptoms

Acute shock and anaemia with the membranes of the mouth ice cold and as white as paper. There is marked abdominal swelling and pain.

Treatment

Emergency surgery. If the highly vascular damaged spleen is not removed quickly, the dog will bleed to death. Its life very much depends on the skill and speed of the veterinary surgeon.

SPLENIC TUMOUR

Symptoms

The dog goes off its food and becomes dull and listless. The membranes of the eye are pasty and pallid *(photo 3)*. The abdomen is enlarged and is painful when pressed.

The diagnosis of a splenic tumour is not easy by any means and even with the aid of X-rays the veterinary surgeon may not be able to specifically determine the tumour site until he opens up the abdomen.

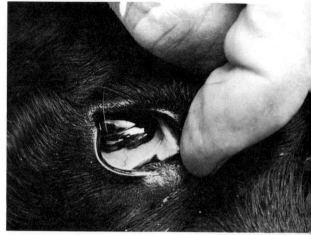

3

Treatment

Surgical removal of the spleen *(photo 4)*. This operation can be spectacularly successful. The spleen is apparently not essential to normal life as the liver is. After a comparatively short convalescent period the dog will return to complete normality and live out its full life span quite happily.

4

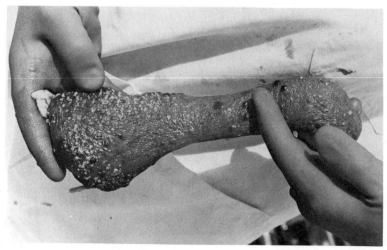

L

43
Lymph and the Lymphatics

LYMPH IS a watery fluid similar to blood plasma. It plays a vital part in conveying nutrients from the blood to the tissues.

Certain parts of the body such as the cornea (front portion of the eye, *photo 1*) and cartilage depend entirely on lymph for their nourishment.

But perhaps even more important, lymph conveys the waste products via minute vessels similar in structure to small veins to the larger lymphatics which pass quietly in and out of what we call lymphatic glands dotted throughout the body.

The entire system can in many ways be compared to the sewage system of a town. The lymphatics are the pipes and the lymphatic glands the disposal centres.

The lymphatics act by contraction of the muscles during exercise—they have no pumping mechanism like the blood vessels. It is a one-way system from the terminal lymph vessels (which run alongside the capillaries) to the lymphatics (i.e. the larger vessels), then to lymph glands where they discharge their waste. Eventually the lymphatics open into the veins at the root of the neck, restoring purified lymph to the bloodstream. It is a complicated and vital system.

Obviously, therefore, a disease of the lymphatic glands can produce serious and fatal results.

The two killer diseases that appear to favour the lymphatics for travelling are

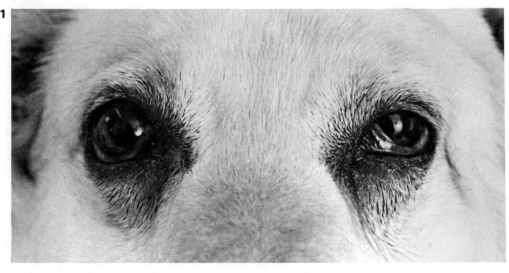
1

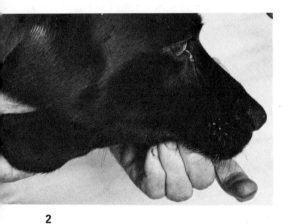

2

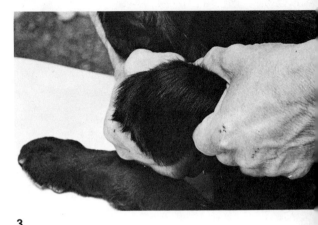

3

tuberculosis and cancer. Because of the
virtual disappearance of the former, the
latter is now the lymphatic disease of
major importance.

Cancer of the Lymphatics

LYMPHOSARCOMA

This can occur in dogs of any age. The
majority of the lymphatic glands and
eventually all of them become cancerous.

Symptoms
The first sign observed by the owner is a
lump or lumps developing under the throat
(photo 2). These lumps vary in size and
are hard and non-painful. Usually the dog
is described as being 'perfectly normal in
every way apart from the lumps'.

The lumps are cancerous lymphatic
glands.

The veterinary surgeon will trace the
other surface lymphatic glands and will
find similar non-painful hard lumps in
most *(photos 3 and 4)*.

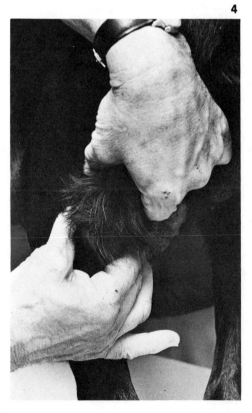

4

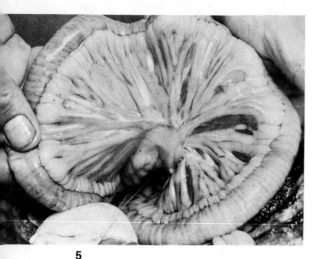

5

Treatment

There is no specific treatment for lympho-sarcoma in animals, radium therapy being economically out of the question.

Since such patients often carry on normally for some time, I advise owners to forget about the lumps unless or until the dog goes off colour.

When the entire tract becomes involved the dog becomes dull and listless, goes off its food and lies about. Painless euthanasia is then indicated.

MESENTERIC LYMPHADENITIS

Comparatively frequently dog cancer starts in the lymphatic glands that run alongside the intestines—called the mesenteric glands *(photo 5)*. When this happens, the condition of mesenteric lymphadenitis develops.

Symptoms

The first signs can resemble very close those of intestinal obstruction (see 'Foreign Body', page 183).

Vomiting, loss in weight and general lack of energy are all typical symptoms.

Diagnosis will require a careful veterinary examination. Usually one or several hard lumps can be felt in the abdomen. X-rays will reveal the extent of spread.

Treatment

Exploratory laparotomy. This means simply opening up the abdomen to have a look. If the spread is localised, the infected glands can be removed. If generalised, the animal is either put quietly to sleep or stitched up *(photo 6)* and returned to the owner for the final decision as to whether to allow the dog to live out the rest of its brief life at least in some discomfort, or to authorise euthanasia.

6

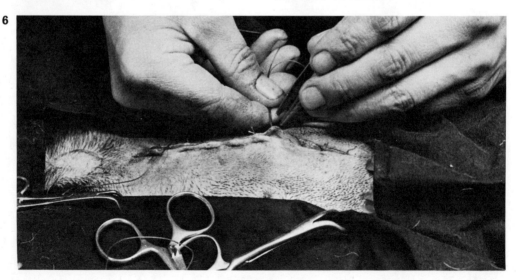

44
The Pancreas

THE PANCREAS is important in all animals but particularly in dogs. It is a small gland rather like a salivary gland and lies in the loop of the duodenum, i.e. the first part of the small intestine.

The greater part of the pancreas is concerned with the production of pancreatic juice containing important salts and enzymes vital to digestion. The pancreatic juice is conveyed to the intestine by two pancreatic ducts.

Dotted through the gland substance are groups of islets which produce insulin and pour it directly into the bloodstream.

Insulin controls the utilisation of sugar by the body and its excretion in the urine.

PANCREATIC DISEASE

Pancreatic disease in the dog *(photo 1)* occurs when the glandular part of the pancreas is not functioning properly and the resultant juice is lacking in enzymes.

Symptoms

Persistent diarrhoea and unthriftiness despite an apparently healthy appetite.

1
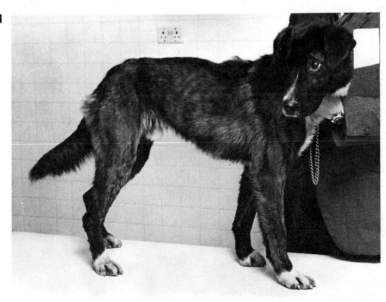

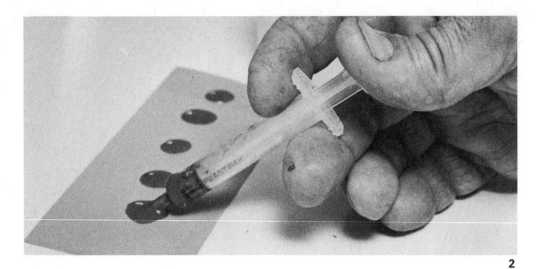

The faeces may not be acutely diarrhoeic—merely sloppy and unformed—but the unthriftiness is a constant feature. In recent years this disease has appeared more frequently, so I would advise all owners to look out for it.

The signs are manifest from an early age—usually during the first nine months of life.

Treatment
The veterinary surgeon will first of all confirm the diagnosis by testing the faeces in the laboratory *(photo 2)*. The test is a simple one and can be carried out within 20–30 minutes.

He will then prescribe capsules or tablets containing the missing enzymes in synthetic form *(photo 3)*.

One capsule is given approximately twenty minutes before each feed and treatment has to be continued for at least three months. After that time many pancreases resume normal activity though in some cases treatment has to be continued throughout the whole of the dog's life.

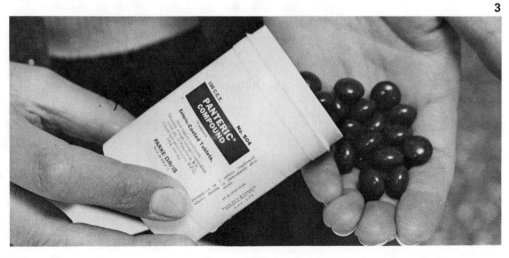

DIABETES

Two types of diabetes occur in dogs: Diabetes mellitus and diabetes insipidus.

DIABETES MELLITUS

This occurs when there is a disturbance or cessation of the production of the insulin. The body sugar, instead of being used to feed the tissues, is excreted in the urine and wasted. Diabetes mellitus, in my experience, occurs most often in bitches.

Symptoms

I have found that these can be variable, but the cardinal features are that the bitch develops an excessive thirst *(photo 4)* and passes excess urine often in large amounts.

The appetite remains good but the condition deteriorates rapidly.

If undetected, the belly becomes dropsical and the dog's energy seems to disappear. There may be occasional vomiting. Later a cataract may develop in one or both eyes.

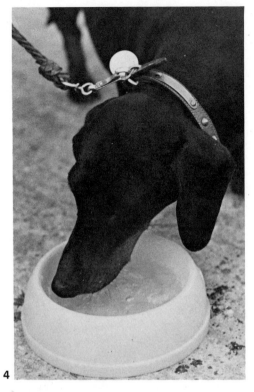

4

Treatment

Whenever the animal develops an excess thirst, get it to a veterinary surgeon immediately, taking with you if possible, a sample of the urine. *(photo 5)*.

The veterinary surgeon will be able to confirm the diagnosis by testing the urine,

5

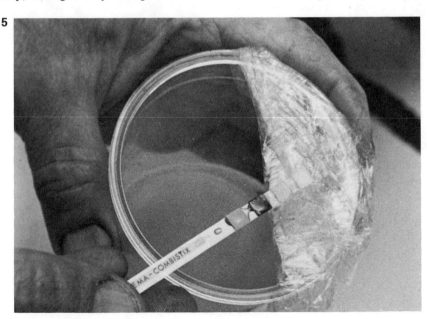

though he will probably also take a blood sample for confirmatory diagnosis *(photo 6)*. If the condition is mild the veterinary surgeon will advise reduction of the carbohydrate intake and will prescribe an oral hypoglycaemic drug.

Most likely, however, he will have to prescribe daily injections of insulin which are the only effective treatment. There will be a trial period before the veterinary surgeon can stabilise the correct daily dosage. I have found this to vary between six and ten units daily depending on the size and weight of the patient *(photo 7)*.

6

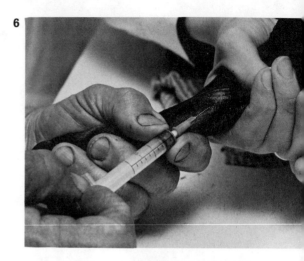

Is Treatment Successful?
Moderately so. I have kept a number of patients going for several years, but only one without developing the cataract.

7

DIABETIC COMA
This occurs when the diabetic patient develops acute hypoglycaemia (shortage of sugar in the body). Obviously, it is more likely to occur when the condition has been undiagnosed, but it can occur during treatment.

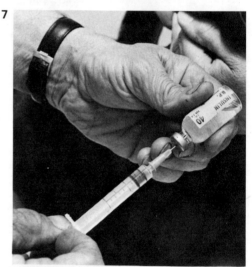

Symptoms
The animal staggers about then goes into a coma *(photo 8)*.

Treatment
Glucose or sugar solution given by the mouth.

8

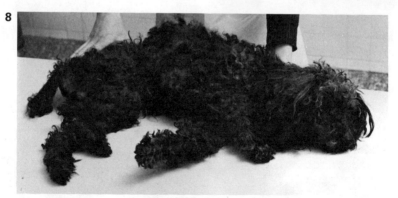

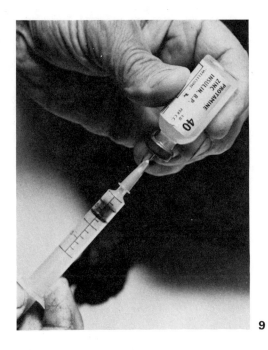

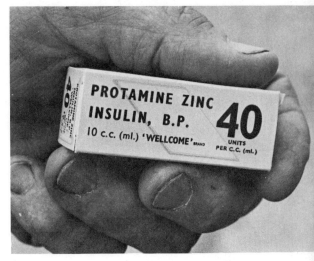

10

9

11

Prevention
Always use insulin containing zinc. I recommend protamine zinc insulin *(photo 9 and 10)*.

DIABETES INSIPIDUS
In this there is no disturbance in insulin production and no urinary sugar excess.

Symptoms
Seen equally in dogs and bitches. Excessive quantities of urine are passed with or without apparent excess drinking (a condition known as Polyuria *(photo 11)*.

No sugar is detected in the urine though the appetite is poor, the coat dull and there is a history of floor-wetting during the night.

Cause
Diabetes Insipidus (Polyuria) can be triggered off by shock or fear, though most of the cases I have seen have followed an acute debilitating disease.

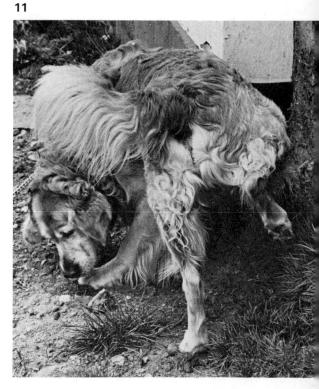

169

Treatment

Confirm the diagnosis by a visit to your veterinary surgeon.

Feed in the mornings only and withhold food and water in the evening.

The veterinary surgeon will probably advise this and at the same time prescribe tranquillisers to control the night incontinence, small doses of modern steroids to improve the appetite, and a general glycerophosphate tonic to restore the dog to normal health. He may inject a hormone called pitressin.

Do Such Cases Recover?

In my experience classic uncomplicated cases of Diabetes Insipidus always recover provided the owner has the nursing patience.

45
Nephritis

NEPHRITIS simply means inflammation of the kidneys. It is one of the commonest and certainly one of the most serious and difficult to treat of all dog conditions, though it affects chiefly ageing dogs *(photo 1)*.

Symptoms
The first sign is usually drinking excess of water and passing excess of urine. The breath may be foul-smelling, though at this stage ulcers are not usually present.

Despite an apparently healthy appetite the dog will rapidly lose condition.

If untreated, the patient may start to vomit especially in the morning.

In advanced cases vomiting becomes incessant especially after drinking water. The breath is foul-smelling; ulcers appear in the mouth *(photo 2)* and the dog goes completely off its food and off its legs.

1

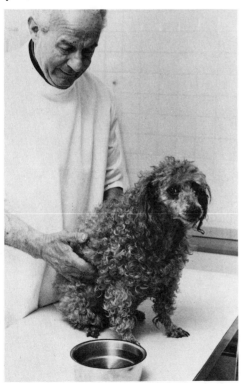

2

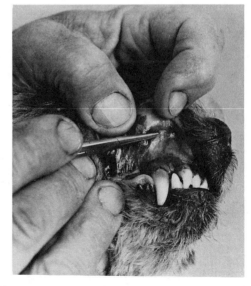

Cause

Certain bacteria, though the specific cause is often unknown.

Predisposing causes—chills. Nephritis often develops in old Poodles that are clipped during the winter—a foolish habit started by convention and perpetuated by the Poodle parlours.

Treatment

Veterinary attention is required urgently and the earlier treatment is applied the better the chance of success.

The kidney is such a complicated organ that any damage is likely to be irreparable. Treatment is aimed at arresting the damage and allowing the remaining kidney tissue to enlarge and compensate for that lost. If infection is suspected, broad spectrum antibiotics are prescribed both orally and by injection *(photo 3)*.

The veterinary surgeon will test the urine and blood and prescribe accordingly.

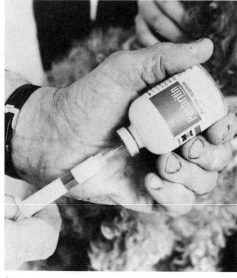

3

Do Nephritis Cases Recover?

If due to infection and caught reasonably early, then nephritis cases can be apparently completely cured by modern drugs.

Can It Be Prevented?

Certainly the traditional six-week clipping of Poodles in the winter time should be banned completely—it is a crazy routine. Again and again I see women draped in furs in a bitterly cold mid winter evening bringing in a freshly clipped shivering, miserable little Poodle in the early stages of nephritis, fibrositis or gastro-enteritis. Such a routine is stupid—Poodles should NEVER be clipped in the winter, no matter how untidy their coats may become.

46
Cystitis

CYSTITIS simply means inflammation of the bladder *(photo 1)*. In my experience it occurs more frequently in bitches than in dogs.

Cause
Bacteria or fungi which gain entrance to the bladder via the urethra (i.e. the opening into the vagina). Again, chills and cold are predisposing factors.

One other cause is the presence of stones (see 'Stones in Bladder', page 175).

Symptoms
The outstanding symptom is repeated urination with night incontinence *(photo 2)*. The bitch may or may not run a temperature but the appetite is capricious and vomiting can occur. Blood may or may not be present in the urine.

Treatment
A visit to the veterinary surgeon immediately; if possible, take a urine sample with you.

The veterinary surgeon will send the urine to a laboratory for cultural examination (or culture it in his own lab—I usually do).

He will probably prescribe a specific urinary antibiotic and/or antiseptic and will X-ray to make sure stones are not present.

Prevention
Again avoid trimming of the coat in winter.

Prognosis
Cystitis usually responds very well to treatment with the cure often a permanent one.

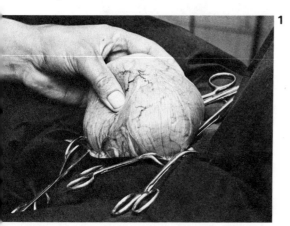

1

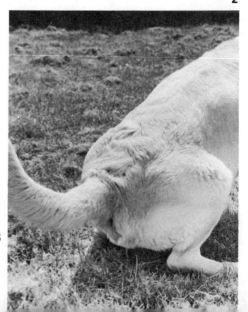

2

47

Stones in the Kidneys, Bladder and Urethra

STONES IN THE KIDNEYS

THESE ARE formed from certain varying compositions of minerals and salts (phosphates, urates, oxalates, etc) but exactly how or why their formation takes place has not as yet been discovered *(photo 1)*.

Symptoms

It is my experience that kidney stones in the dog rarely cause apparent trouble, though this may be due to the difficulty of diagnosis.

In the comparatively few cases I have seen, the history has been one of bouts of acute pain for no apparent reason, with the dog howling piteously for varying periods.

Diagnosis

Diagnosis has only been possible by X-ray.

Treatment

Most kidney stones, if left alone, will pass from the kidneys down through the ureter to the bladder.

Where the stone is large, however, and especially where it is occupying most of the pelvis of the kidney (i.e. the portion where the ureter joins), surgical removal may be attempted. For this job a thorough knowledge of the anatomy of the kidney is required.

1

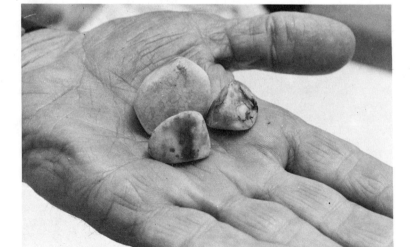

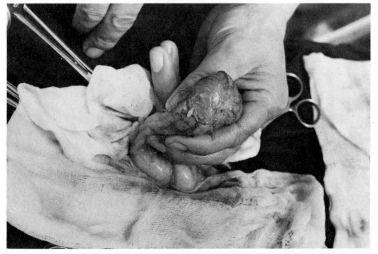

2

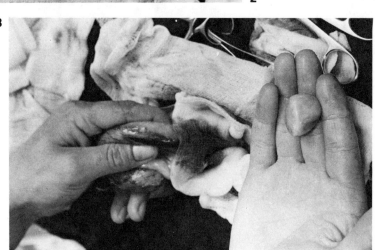

3

STONES IN THE BLADDER

It is when the stones are in the bladder that typical symptoms most often appear *(photo 2)*.

Symptoms

The signs are similar to those seen in cystitis but blood is very often present in the urine. X-rays will confirm the diagnosis.

Treatment

The only satisfactory treatment is surgical removal. This operation is usually completely successful *(photo 3)*.

Prevention

Unfortunately it is not possible to anticipate the formation of bladder stones though they appear to form more frequently in certain parts of the country, no doubt because of the varying composition of the water supplies.

Once the stones have been removed, however, it is possible to have them analysed and to prescribe a simple drug which will help to prevent them reforming.

A recent analysis for example was as follows:

Ammonium urate	10%
Oxalate	5%
Phosphates	85%

As a prevention I have prescribed a daily dose of five grams of sodium acid phosphate (aqueous solution).

STONES IN URETHRA

This syndrome is seen almost exclusively in male dogs, the simple reason being that the urethra of the dog is very much longer than in the bitch.

The stones travel down from the bladder and block the urethra usually at the beginning of the os penis (bone of the penis) *(see diagram)*.

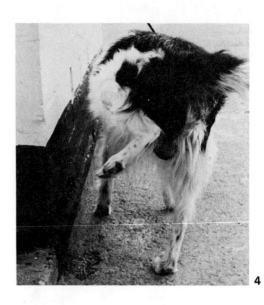

4

Diagram of bladder, kidneys, ureter and urethra.

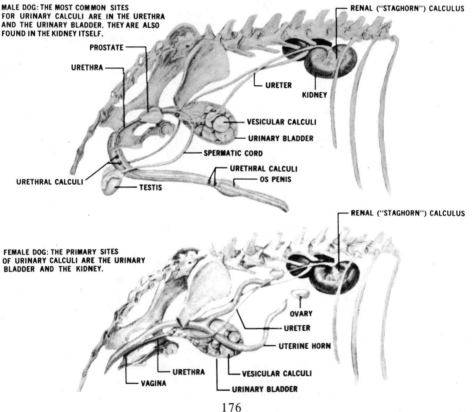

MALE DOG: THE MOST COMMON SITES FOR URINARY CALCULI ARE IN THE URETHRA AND THE URINARY BLADDER. THEY ARE ALSO FOUND IN THE KIDNEY ITSELF.

PROSTATE

URETHRA

RENAL ("STAGHORN") CALCULUS

URETER

KIDNEY

VESICULAR CALCULI

URINARY BLADDER

SPERMATIC CORD

URETHRAL CALCULI

URETHRAL CALCULI

OS PENIS

TESTIS

RENAL ("STAGHORN") CALCULUS

FEMALE DOG: THE PRIMARY SITES OF URINARY CALCULI ARE THE URINARY BLADDER AND THE KIDNEY.

OVARY

URETER

UTERINE HORN

URETHRA

VESICULAR CALCULI

VAGINA

URINARY BLADDER

176

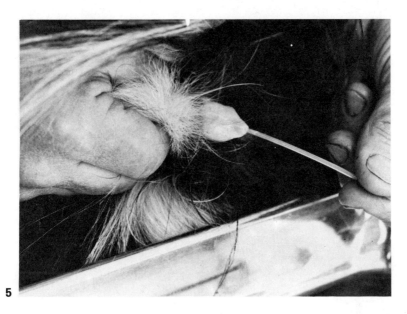

5

Symptoms

The dog repeatedly passes urine either in small jets or in minute drops or else, in advanced cases, continually tries to urinate without success *(photo 4)*.

Treatment

An emergency operation has to be performed so get the dog to the veterinary surgeon as quickly as possible.

The veterinary surgeon will pass a catheter *(photo 5)* to locate the blockage then, under local or general anaesthesia will cut straight down onto the stones and remove them. He will then ensure that the urethra is clear by passing the catheter through into the bladder.

Personally I always X-ray the bladder and kidneys as a routine in all cases of urethral obstruction and usually do a combined cystotomy and urethrotomy (i.e. I remove the stones from the bladder and urethra during the one general anaesthesia).

M

48
The Teeth

THE DOG becomes an adult at nine months and at that age it should have a full mouth of permanent teeth. In fact the majority of dogs have a full set at seven months.

Since there appears to be a general misunderstanding of the dog's dentition, the following photograph *(1)* and table should explain it fully.

Tooth	*Eruption (Temporary)* (weeks)	*Change to Permanent* (months)
Incisor 1 (1_1)	4–5	
Incisor 2 (1_2)	4–5	4–5
Incisor 3 (1_3)	4	
Canine (C)	3–4	4–5
Premolar 1 (P_1)	4–5	
Premolar 2 (P_2)	4–5	5–6
Premolar 3 (P_3)	3–4	
Premolar 4 (P_4)	3–4	
Molar 1 (M_1)		4
Molar 2 (M_2)		Upper 5–6 Lower $4\frac{1}{2}$–5
Molar 3		6–7

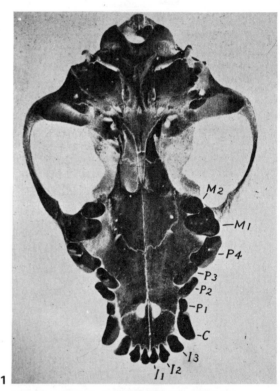

1

Tooth Structure (*Diagram A*)

Each tooth has a portion covered with enamel—the 'crown'; a portion covered with cement—the 'root'; and a line of union between these two parts known as the neck.

The tooth consists of four tissues. In the middle is the "pulp", occupying the "pulp cavity". It is soft and well supplied with blood vessels and nerves. Its function is to nourish the tooth and form the "dentine".

The "dentine" forms the greater part of the tooth. It is hard and yellowish in colour, and is surrounded in the crown by the "enamel", and the root by the "cement".

The root of the tooth is embedded in a cavity in the jaw bone known as "the alveolus".

Since dogs are carnivores, their teeth are adapted for hunting. They do not keep food in their mouths for very long.

Their large hooked canine teeth are used to seize or transfix their food, and their side and back teeth are adapted more for shearing than grinding.

Since tooth troubles in the domestic dog are very common I shall deal with them in simple question and answer form.

What Causes Discoloured Teeth?
A deposition of a soft deposit known as 'plaque' which forms on the enamel surface of the tooth, particularly at the 'neck' or gum margin *(photo 2)*.

Plaque is produced by the combined action of bacteria, saliva, putrefying foodstuffs and certain enzymes.

What Causes Tartar?
Once plaque is established, mineral salts are deposited on it from the saliva producing what is commonly known as 'tartar'—the scientific name being 'calculus' *(photo 3)*.

Diagram A

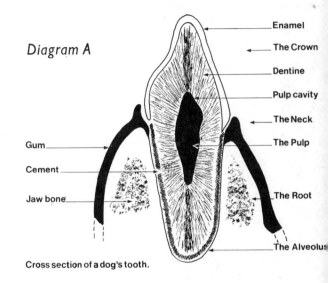

Cross section of a dog's tooth.

Naturally the longer the condition is left untreated, the thicker and more offensive it becomes.

What Causes Bad Breath?
The most common cause is the deposition of plaque and tartar, but persistent bad

2   **3**

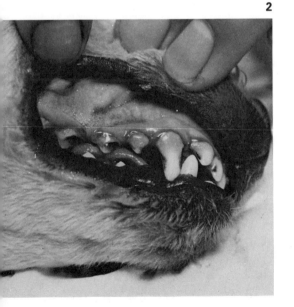

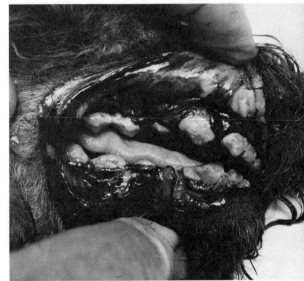

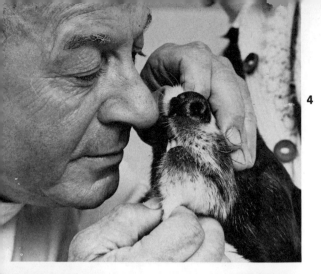

4

breath is often observed in clean-mouthed dogs *(photo 4)*. Such cases are due to digestive disturbances and can be treated successfully by your veterinary surgeon.

Does Bad Breath do Any Harm?
If due to plaque or tartar, both these lead to separation of the teeth from the gums and eventual tooth decay. If due to digestive disturbances, the only harm is the unpleasant mouth odour.

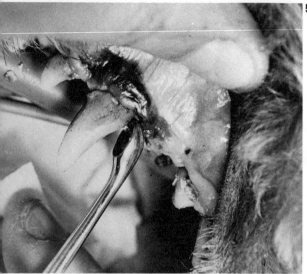

5

What Can be Done?
The obvious answer is a regular visit to your veterinary surgeon. Six monthly visits are advised for human teeth. I'd suggest a twelve-month inspection for dogs.

Plaque and tartar can easily be dealt with, though in both cases an anaesthetic may be required *(photo 5)*.

THE CARNASSIAL TOOTH
The only tooth in the dog which produces a special problem is what we call the 'carnassial' tooth *(photo 6)*.

The carnassial is situated one on either side of the upper jaw. It is a very powerful tooth with double roots which are subject to decay in ageing dogs.

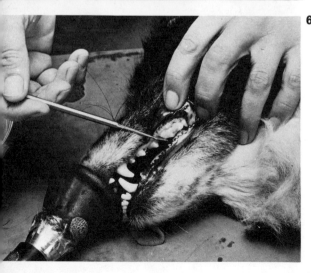

6

The first sign of trouble is usually a swelling on the side of the dog's upper jaw underneath the eye.

The dog usually shows signs of discomfort or pain—tending to go off his food or lie about shivering occasionally.

If neglected, the swelling which is in fact an abscess in the sinus or cavity into which the carnassial alveolus extends will eventually burst producing what we call a fistula *(photo 7)*.

Treatment
The offending carnassial tooth must be removed as soon as possible under a general anaesthetic *(photo 8)*.

Can Teeth Disease be Prevented?

The simple answer is yes. A yearly visit to your veterinary surgeon is all that is necessary.

Regular cleaning of the teeth with toothpaste, powder, a mouth wash or antiseptic gel will help tremendously to prevent plaque and tartar, but this is a chore which few pet owners could discipline themselves to.

One routine that does help is the chewing of large bones—a large knuckle bone once a week helps to keep the teeth clean and the dog will enjoy chewing it, *but on no account feed small bones such as those from ham, pork, lamb and poultry. Sharp vertebrae and rib bones are particularly dangerous.* These small bones are liable to lodge in the dog's oesophagus (food pipe) or small intestine and lead to a major operation for their removal.

MOUTH ULCERS

These are seen mainly in dogs where the teeth have been neglected though they can appear independently *(photo 9)*.

Causes

1. Abrasion of the gums and inside of the cheeks by overgrown tartar. This is the commonest cause.
2. Pressure of the canines on the lower lips —seen mainly in the larger loose jowled dogs—Spaniels, Pyrenean Mountain dogs, Bloodhounds, etc.
3. Vitamin deficiency—shortage of vitamin B_1 or vitamin E.
4. Kidney disfunction—mouth ulcers are frequently seen in cases of nephritis.
5. Cancer—what we call a rodent ulcer.

Treatment

At the slightest sign of a mouth ulcer take the dog to a veterinary surgeon immediately. He will diagnose the condition and prescribe the specific treatment.

If the teeth are bad he will scale and clean them.

7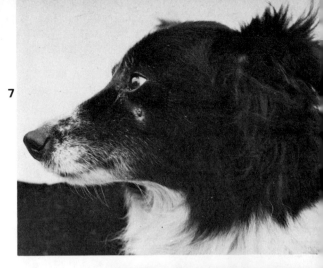

8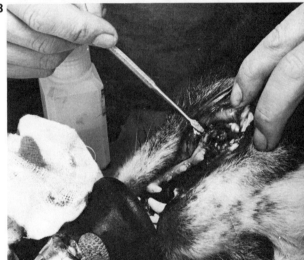

9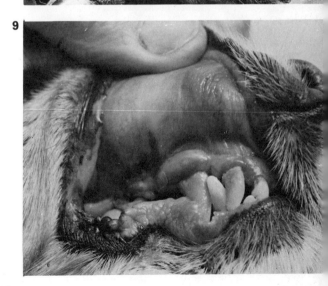

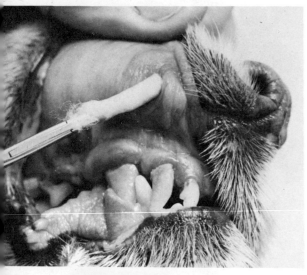

10

The ulcers due to canine pressure he will probably treat by cauterisation *(photo 10)*.

The vitamin deficiency can be corrected and the kidney condition treated.

The rodent ulcer presents a special problem but if seen early can often be surgically removed.

BONE STUCK IN OESOPHAGUS

Symptoms

The puppy or dog will be keen to eat—often ravenous but within seconds will vomit the food back. Water or milk may also be returned, though occasionally they are held down.

11

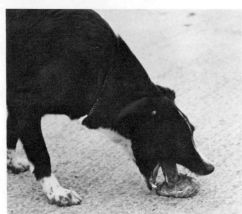

Treatment

An immediate visit to your veterinary surgeon who will confirm the diagnosis by X-ray.

If early on the job, the veterinary surgeon may try vomiting the stomach contents by injecting an emetic *(photo 11)*. The full weight of the stomach contents will often dislodge and bring up the offending portion. I have been successful with this technique on a number of occasions.

If this fails, he will probably try removing the object with the help of an oesophagoscope or probe.

12

It has been my experience that if vomiting the stomach contents does not dislodge, the obstruction then surgery is usually necessary.

Unfortunately the bone is usually lodged in the lower part of the oesophagus and this means going in through the stomach or through the chest.

Probably the most spectacularly successful operation I have personally performed was the removal, through the chest, of a fish hook which was lodged in the thoracic portion of the oesophagus of a small Jack Russell Terrier.

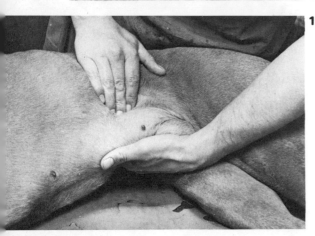

FOREIGN BODY LODGED IN INTESTINES

A natural follow-up to the above ailment is the case of what we call a "foreign body"—it could be a bone or a stone.

History
The condition of "foreign body" is most commonly seen in puppies or dogs which chase stones or sticks thrown by their indulgent owners. Many dogs do this by instinct, especially those bred for retrieving.

It has been my experience that most cases of "foreign body" in the intestines are due to swallowing stones, though I have removed portions of sticks, plastic toys, rubber balls and transfixed needles, and of course the odd small bone which has managed to get past the base of the oesophagus *(photo 12)*.

Perhaps the most interesting case I remember was a Labrador which the owner described as 'making a rattling noise' when it walked. An X-ray revealed a mass of rounded stones in the stomach—ten there proved to be.

So long as the stones remain in the stomach they cause little trouble. The symptoms appear when one lodges in the intestine—usually the small intestine.

Symptoms
The earliest sign is vomiting some time after eating, usually within an hour.

After several vomiting attacks the dog refuses to eat or drink, it looks miserable and dejected; the inside of its mouth becomes cold and clammy. The dog stops passing motions. In many cases these are the signs presented to us.

Treatment
The veterinary surgeon will confirm his diagnosis by X-ray and will operate immediately *(photo 13)*.

Invariably the portion of the bowel

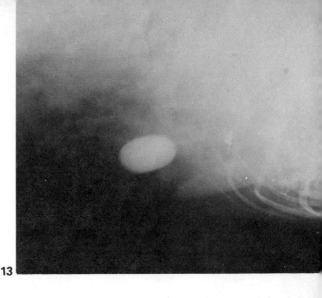

13

where the foreign body is lodged is discoloured and damaged and the surgeon has to remove the object through part of the healthy bowel a little beyond the obstruction. This ensures quicker and better healing *(photo 14)*.

After-Care
The veterinary surgeon will instruct on this but it usually comprises liquids only for two or three days, then soft sloppy feeds for at least three days afterwards.

Is the Operation a Success?
Provided the case is seen reasonably early the success rate is very high. In fact I have seen spectacular recoveries in many advanced cases.

14

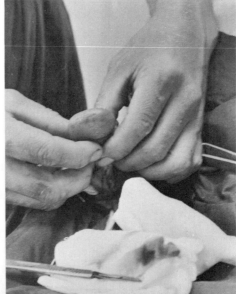

49
The Eye

THE COMMON conditions occurring in the dog's eye are:

1. Conjunctivitis.
2. Corneal Opacity.
3. Glaucoma.
4. Misfunction of the Harderian Gland in the Third Eyelid.
5. Retinal Atrophy.
6. Cataract.
7. Blindness.
8. (a) Entropion, (b) Ectropion.
9. Blocked Tear Duct.
10. Luxation (dislocation) of the Eyeball.

CONJUNCTIVITIS

Conjunctivitis is an inflammation of the Conjunctiva, which is the membrane that covers the front of the eye *(photo 1)*. This membrane lines the insides of both upper and lower eyelids and is reflected on to the front of the eyeball. The centre portion is transparent to allow light into the cavity of the eye, and is richly supplied with nerves.

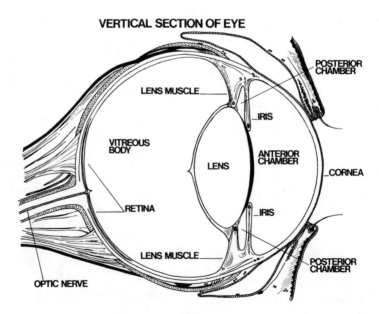

VERTICAL SECTION OF EYE

LENS MUSCLE

POSTERIOR CHAMBER

IRIS

VITREOUS BODY

ANTERIOR CHAMBER

LENS

CORNEA

RETINA

IRIS

LENS MUSCLE

POSTERIOR CHAMBER

OPTIC NERVE

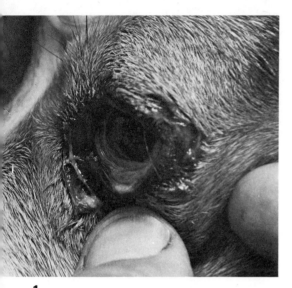

1

Causes

Injuries, infection, and foreign bodies such as dust, sand, pollen, seeds, lime, pieces of chaff, flies, etc.

The direct cause of the inflammation is the activity of the germs which are already present in the eye or which may be blown into it from the air.

Symptoms

The first sign is usually a running eye and a tendency to keep it closed *(photo 2)*. If you open the eye, you will see that it is swollen and red. If untreated, a thicker discharge develops in about 12 hours followed by pus the following day. If still untreated, the purulent discharge marks

2

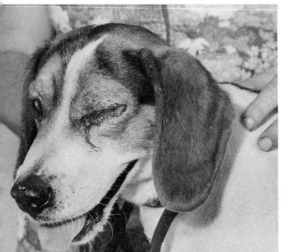

the hair around the eye and if left there will blister the skin.

Treatment

First of all, soak a piece of cotton wool in warm water or saline (half a level teaspoonful of salt to half a pint of warm water). With this clean up the discharge round the eye and search for a foreign body. Needless to say, this is not always easy and it is probably better to take the dog immediately to a veterinary surgeon.

If you are lucky enough to be able to remove a foreign body, a thorough bathing with the warm saline solution will probably clear the condition up. The best way to bathe is merely to open the eye and squeeze the cotton wool which has been soaked in the saline solution. The drops will then wash the eye out *(photo 3)*.

If the conjunctivitis persists, then a veterinary surgeon should be consulted at once since the condition could become chronic and lead to deep-seated infection, ulceration and even blindness.

CORNEAL OPACITY

The technical name for this is keratitis

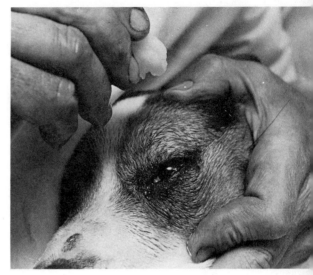

3

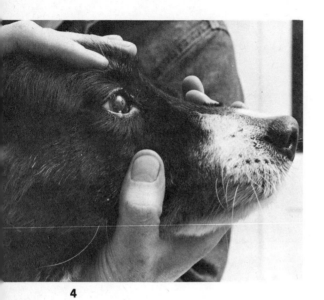

4

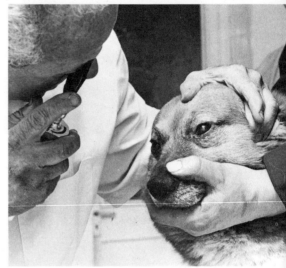

5

(photo 4). The condition is usually described as "a film over the eye". The surface of the cornea, i.e. the central portion of the eye, instead of remaining transparent becomes opaque due to its nourishing fluid called lymph coagulating.

Unlike practically all other parts of the body, the cornea is not nourished by blood, for if it were light could not pass through to the deeper parts of the eye. There are tiny spaces between the cells which compose it and in these spaces there flows clear lymph.

Cause
Inflammation of the cornea (i.e. keratitis). This may be caused by injuries, kicks, blows, running into objects in the dark, etc. Also any one of the foreign bodies mentioned in conjunctivitis can produce a keratitis. It can be caused by the presence of roundworm larvae in the eyes or by draughts. Another cause is entropion, i.e. a turning-in of the eyelids (see 'Entropion', page 190).

Symptoms
In the early stages the condition is indistinguishable from conjunctivitis. When

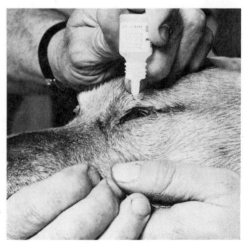

6

the eye is examined the surface of the cornea appears dull or blueish. If untreated, it becomes opaque and pus forms in the eye *(photo 5)*. If still untreated, ulceration develops.

Treatment
Corneal opacity is a serious condition and should always be treated by a veterinary surgeon *(photo 6)*. He will establish the cause and prescribe a specific cure.

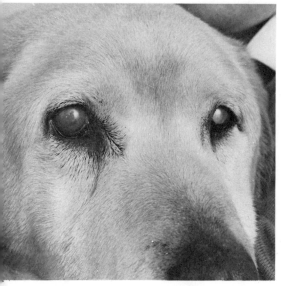

7

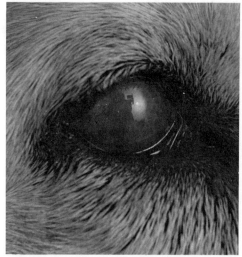

8

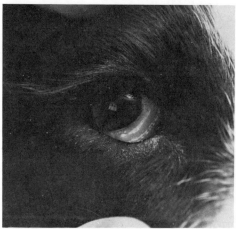

9

GLAUCOMA

Glaucoma occurs when there is obstruction to the drainage system of the eye *(photo 7)*. This leads to an excess of fluid in the eyeball and causes the affected eye to swell up.

Cause
The cause is unknown.

Symptoms
The early signs are identical to those seen in conjunctivitis and keratitis but the diagnostic feature is the bulging of the affected eye with a clouding over of the entire eye surface *(photo 8)*.

Treatment
Very much a job for your veterinary surgeon. Personally I perform an operation which involves making a permanent small hole in the cornea through which the excess fluid drains. If this operation is not successful, the eye may have to be removed.

MISFUNCTION OF HARDERIAN GLAND

The Harderian gland is a small gland situated in the third eyelid in the corner of the dog's eye. A blockage of its ducts or an injury produces a disfunction of the gland and causes it to enlarge *(photo 9)*.

Symptoms
A reddish lump appears in the corner of the eye on the third eyelid.

187

Treatment
Cortisone drops should be tried for a week (your veterinary surgeon will supply these), but if the swelling persists the reddish lump will have to be removed surgically. This operation is very successful and leaves no permanent damage.

RETINAL ATROPHY
Also known as progressive retinal atrophy "night blindness" *(photo 10)*.

Cause
This is a hereditary condition first seen in the Irish Red Setter but now fairly common in a number of breeds including the Poodle.

The retina, i.e. the part of the eye which receives the pictures from outside, undergoes a progressive wasting causing impaired vision which invariably tends to get worse.

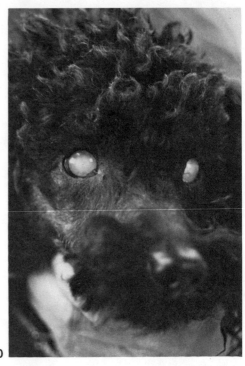

10

Symptoms
The dog's pupil dilates widely even in daylight giving a staring expression. The eyes are obviously defective and at night or in poor light the dog stumbles into lamp posts and other objects in its path.

During full daylight it may appear to see quite well. The disease usually starts to develop when the dog is three to five months old.

Treatment
There is none. The affected puppy or dog becomes gradually more and more blind.

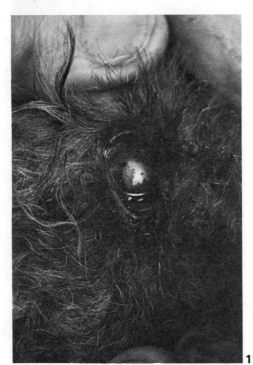

11

CATARACT
Cataract occurs when the lens of the eye loses its transparency *(photo 11)*.

Cause
Any condition which interferes with the nutrition of the lens, e.g. glaucoma,

injuries, etc. The cataract may be congenital but it is usually associated with old age.

Symptoms
The congenital cases are blind from an early age and the lack of transparency in the lens can be detected by examining the eye with an opthalmascope. Usually, however, it does not appear until the dog is between nine and ten years old.

Treatment
The only treatment is the removal of the lens. However, since it is not as yet possible to fit contact lenses to dogs, the operation is only moderately successful. It improves the vision slightly by allowing the dog to appreciate objects at a certain fixed distance.

BLINDNESS
Blindness in the dog may be congenital but is usually associated with some disease, poison or deficiency *(photo 12)*.

Causes
1. Disease of the retina, optic nerve or brain.
2. Poisoning by certain plants, e.g. rape or by lead.
3. Glaucoma, dislocation of the lens or cataract.
4. Deficiency of vitamin A.

Treatment
Obviously it is essential to find out the cause of the blindness before attempting treatment and this is very much a matter for your veterinary surgeon.

12

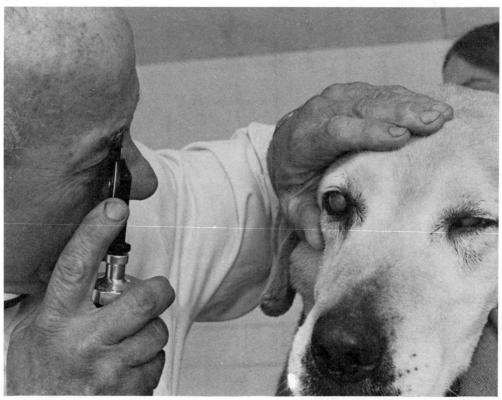

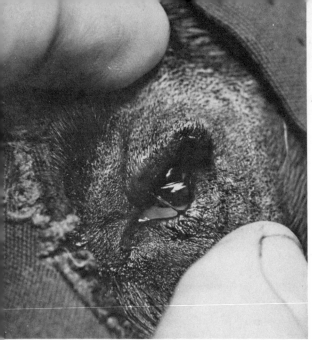

ENTROPION

Entropion is a turning-in of the eyelids, usually the lower eyelid *(photo 13)*. The condition may be congenital.

Symptoms

The dog shows obvious signs of discomfort, continually blinking its eye which discharges profusely. If neglected, the turned-in eyelid produces a keratitis, corneal opacity and ulceration.

Treatment

The veterinary surgeon will perform a comparatively simple operation aimed at turning the eyelids back into their normal position *(photo 14)*.

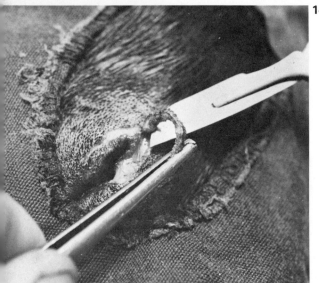

14

ECTROPION

In this condition one or both eyelids are pouched outwards so that the conjunctiva is exposed *(photo 15)*. It is seen particularly in Bloodhounds and St. Bernards.

Symptoms

There is a tendency for the eyes to continually water and this usually forms a black mark down the side of the dog's cheeks. The pink or red conjunctiva is clearly visible.

Treatment

Ectropion is accepted as normal in Bloodhounds and St. Bernards but when it occurs in other breeds a surgical operation is again required. This time a portion of the conjunctiva is removed instead of a

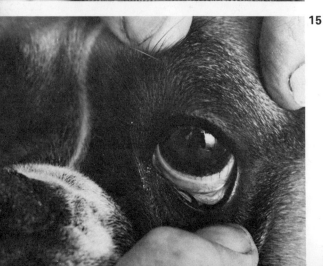

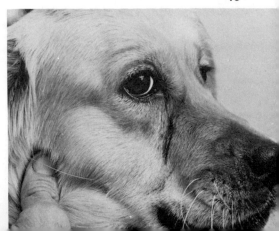

part of the skin of the eyelid. The opera- **18**
tion is usually successful.

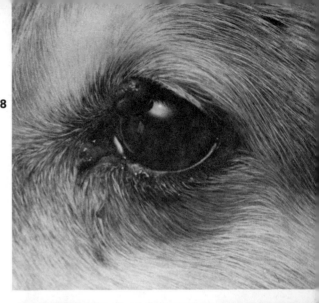

BLOCKED TEAR DUCT

Symptoms
This condition scientifically described as
Epiphora leads to a continual discharge
of tears from the eye *(photo 16)*.

Causes
Obstruction in the lacrimal duct which
normally drains from the eye to the nasal
cavity. It can occur secondary to conjunctivitis or any one of the other eye **19**
conditions.

Treatment
It is usually possible to clear the blockage
in the tear duct by probing with a piece of
firm nylon suture material or by syringing
the duct through under pressure *(photo 17)*.
This requires a general anaesthetic and
should only be attempted by a veterinary
surgeon.

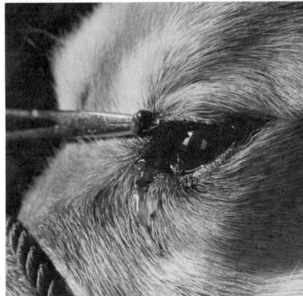

WART ON EYELID
This is not uncommon. As the wart increases in size it irritates the eye surface
producing a keratitis *(photo 18)*.

Treatment
Surgical removal under local or general
anaesthesia *(photo 19)*. Cauterisation of
the wart base usually prevents a recur- **20**
rence *(photo 20)*.

17

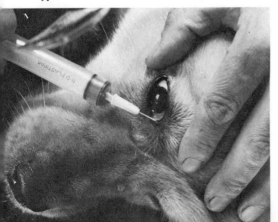

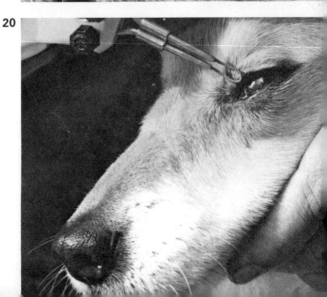

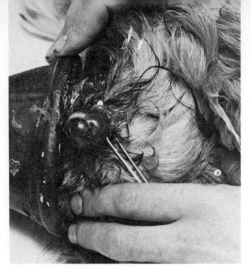

21

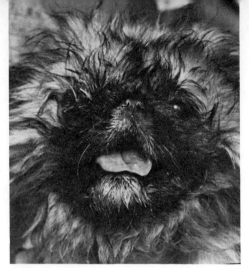

22

LUXATION (DISLOCATION) OF THE EYEBALL

This is most commonly seen in the Pekinese *(photo 21)*.

It is caused usually by another dog or the owner gripping the Peke by the scruff of the neck.

Treatment

This is an emergency. The quicker you get the patient to a veterinary surgeon, the better. He will do his utmost to replace the eyeball in the socket *(photo 22)* and suture the lids to hold it in position, removing the sutures in 10–12 days.

Where the luxation is long standing, or when the eye is badly damaged, the entire eye has to be removed *(photo 23)*.

DRY EYE

Thought to be due to deficient tear production, secondary to a virus or bacterial infection of the lacrimal glands.

Symptoms

In the early stages the signs are identical to conjunctivitis, namely a catarrhal discharge and a running eye. However, true dry eye does not respond satisfactorily to treatment and a degree of keratitis develops.

Whenever kerato-conjunctivitis fails to respond to treatment, dry eye should always be suspected *(photo 24)*.

Treatment

Very much a job for your veterinary surgeon. He will prescribe artificial tear drops and antibiotic ointment. Where the condition persists for months, as it usually does, the veterinary surgeon may perform a parotid duct transplant.

23

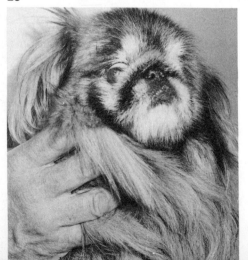

24

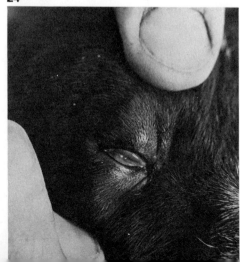

50
The Ear

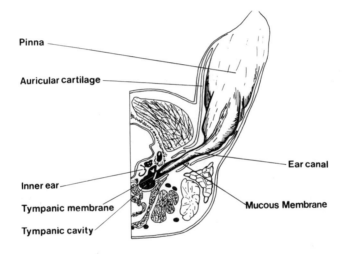

Pinna

Auricular cartilage

Inner ear

Tympanic membrane

Tympanic cavity

Ear canal

Mucous Membrane

VERTICAL SECTION OF THE EAR

IN ORDER TO understand ear conditions it is necessary to have a simple knowledge of the auditory anatomy. The above sketch illustrates this adequately. The entire ear cavity is lined by a membrane which we call mucous membrane.

Diseases of the Ear

Practically all ear conditions in dogs can be treated with complete success if they are caught early enough *(photo 1)*. Therefore at the slightest sign of irritation or discomfort a veterinary surgeon should be con-

sulted immediately. Once the condition becomes established, a cure can be protracted, difficult or even impossible. Certainly

1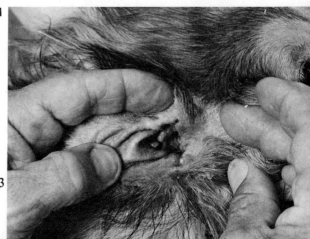

N

there is a tendency for the mucous membrane to become ulcerated.

CANKER

Canker is the general name given to any inflammation of the lining of the external ear.

2

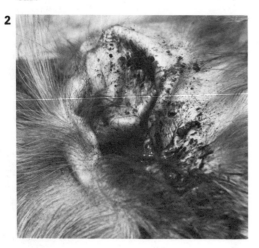

Causes
1. An excess of wax *(photo 2)*.
2. Reddening or eczema of the mucous membrane due in many cases to feeding excess of carbohydrate (a meal allergy).
3. Infection secondary to eczema.
4. Parasites (ear mange).

Symptoms
The first sign is usually a shaking of the head or a rubbing of the offending ear on

3

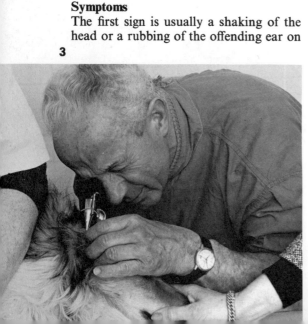

4

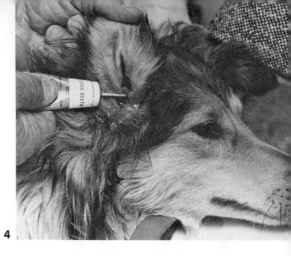

the floor or against the furniture. Examination of the external ear may show an excess of wax or a severe reddening and there may be an offensive smell. The veterinary surgeon can usually establish the precise cause by examining with an auroscope *(photo 3)*.

Treatment
Since the entire ear apparatus is extremely delicate and irreplaceable, it is always best to have the ear treated by a veterinary surgeon.

If excess wax is the cause, he will probably syringe the ear out, clean the cavity (taking great care not to damage the mucous membrane) and prescribe an antibiotic and an anti-inflammatory agent *(photo 4)*.

In chronic cases, especially where ulceration is present, after a thorough cleansing of the cavity it may be necessary to cauterise the ulcers with a five or ten per cent solution of silver nitrate before prescribing the treatment *(photo 5)*.

5

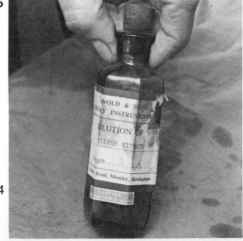

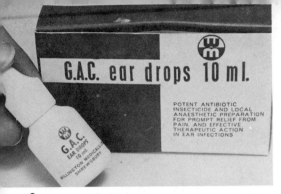

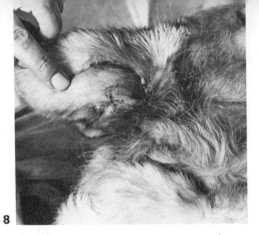

6 If the canker is due to otodectic mange, then drops prescribed will contain Gammexane, a powerful anti-parasitic agent *(photo 6)*.

As mentioned above, treatment should always be supervised by a veterinary surgeon. Cotton wool should never be forced down the ears since the rough fibres damage the mucous membrane and predispose to infection; nor should any powder be introduced since this has the same damaging effect.

In long-standing cases where infection persists despite treatment, a successful operation can be performed. This surgery, called Zepp's operation, comprises opening up the ear channel down to the base to provide perfect drainage *(photo 7)*.

FOREIGN BODIES IN EAR

In the smaller breeds particularly, hay or grass seeds, gravel, stones or glass splinters may get into the ear cavity.

Symptoms
The irritation is excessive and often the dog literally "goes mad" with discomfort and pain.

Treatment
Very much a matter for your veterinary surgeon who will identify the cause with

8 his auroscope and if necessary give an anaesthetic to ensure complete removal.

HAEMATOMA

A haematoma is a collection of bruised blood. When it occurs on the ear, it does so between the cartilage and the skin on the inside *(photo 8)*. It is seen mostly in the larger breed of dogs.

Cause
The common cause is scratching the ear due to one of the conditions described under canker but it can be caused by a direct injury.

Treatment
Again very much a job for your veterinary surgeon. He will make a long elliptical opening on the inside of the flap, remove the contents and suture the wound in such a way that the collection cannot reform *(photo 9)*.

7

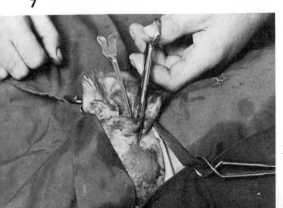

9

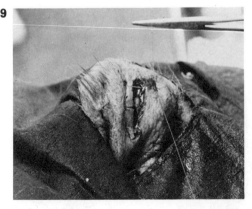

WOUNDS

One of the most difficult conditions to treat in any dog is a wound on the ear flap because of the persistent shaking of the head and the comparative poor blood supply to the part *(photo 10)*. Both make healing a slow process.

10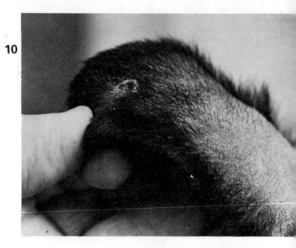

Cause

Usually a bite from another dog or a tear by barbed wire or glass. One of the worst cases I had to treat recently was where a dog had jumped through a greenhouse window.

Treatment

As a first-aid measure a thick wad of cotton wool should be put over the wound and the ear flap bandaged flat as illustrated *(photo 11)*. The patient should then be taken to a veterinary surgeon who will probably suture or cauterize the wound.

11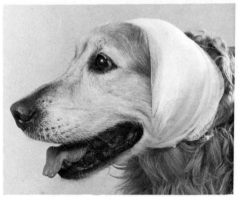

TUMOURS

Often as a result of infection small warts or tumours appear in a dog's ear. The only satisfactory treatment is surgical removal.

51
The Nervous System

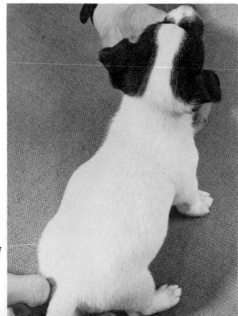

1

AS IN HUMANS the dog's nervous
system is complex and finely developed
and any disfunction, no matter how slight
is quickly manifest. The nervous problems
we have to cope with in practice are:

1. Fits.
2. Chorea.
3. Cerebral Haemorrhage.
4. Peripheral Neuritis.
5. Hysteria.
6. Radial Paralysis.

FITS
Convulsions with the dog kicking and
frothing at the mouth and apparently
unconscious *(photo 1)*. The fit may last
for only a few seconds and often occurs
when the dog is sleeping.

Cause
Mostly epilepsy, the precise cause of which
is not fully understood.

The earliest age occurrence is when
pups are cutting their teeth at two to six
months especially when they are heavily
infested with worms—round or tape. The
infested pup is usually pot-bellied *(photo
2)*.

2

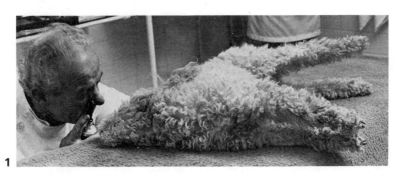

Later the epilepsy can be due to shock, fear, injuries, sexual excitement, pain or stress, e.g. after operations or whelping.

Large feeds of liver and sudden changes of temperature can trigger off an attack.

The most difficult and persistent epileptic fits to treat often appear to have no specific trigger factor and they may be hereditary or the result of brain damage due to a head injury.

Fits, or course are a feature of nervous distemper (see 'Distemper', page 84).

Treatment

As a first-aid measure put the dog in a quiet dark room, surround with cushions and cover over with a blanket, then leave it absolutely alone.

When the dog appears to be completely recovered take it to your veterinary surgeon. He will do his best to ascertain and remove the cause and will probably prescribe one of two drugs, viz. Mysoline (ICI) or Largactil (M & B).

CHOREA

In dogs this appears almost exclusively as a secondary symptom of canine distemper. In humans a similar condition is known as 'St. Vitus's Dance'.

Cause

Damage to the central nervous system as a result of a virus or bacterial infection.

Symptoms

Persistent and apparently uncontrollable twitching of individual or groups of muscles starting usually in the head or one leg *(photo 3)*.

The twitching may spread throughout the whole body. Fits and paralysis often develop.

Treatment

Chorea is a serious and incurable condi-

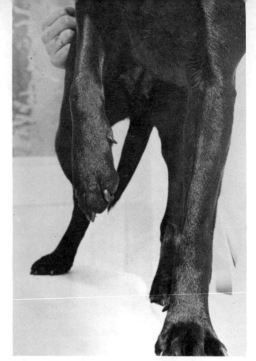

3

tion and the most that one can hope for is that it will not get any worse.

Concentrate on building the animal's strength up with good feeding and an abundance of vitamins.

The veterinary surgeon will prescribe calcium salts and parathyroid extract with or without sedatives. I have 'cured' many cases of chorea, but the twitching has persisted for the rest of the animal's life.

When fits or paralysis set in the case is hopeless and euthanasia is indicated.

CEREBRAL HAEMORRHAGE

Often known as 'a stroke' and seen mainly in older dogs.

Cause

Rupture of one of the small blood vessels in the brain.

Symptoms

Sudden loss of power in one or more limbs. The dog may be completely paralysed though perfectly conscious. There is often a history of staggering and falling about

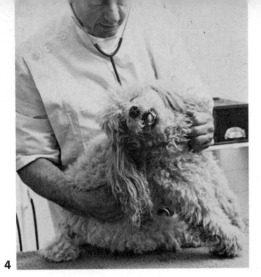

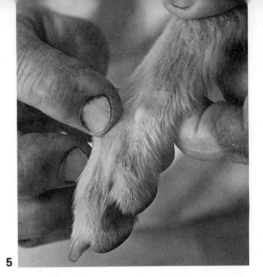

and the head may loll to one side *(photo 4)*.

Treatment

Treatment is not by any means hopeless but it requires great patience and application by the owner: such owners are few and far between. However, with the help of such an owner I cured an eight-year-old Alsatian which was completely paralysed for 14 weeks.

The full credit belonged to the owners who manipulated and massaged the legs for several hours each day to prevent muscular atrophy (wasting) and fed the animal as though it was a child.

Medical treatment comprises anticoagulants, steroids, vitamins and continual hope that other haemorrhages don't occur.

Success depends entirely on nature removing the blood clot.

PERIPHERAL NEURITIS

This means inflammation of the nerve endings *(photo 5)*.

Cause

Often obscure though it may develop secondary to an injury, a scald, or a patch of eczema.

Symptoms

These are localised, the central nervous system being apparently normal.

The dog will bite incessantly usually at a rounded area on a leg or foot; the area may become raw and ulcerated.

Treatment

Tranquillisers combined with painting the area with a noxious-tasting substance such as Friars Balsam. I have found a successful local application to be chloramphenicol and gentian violet in aerosol form *(photo 6)*.

Sometimes the affected area may have to be dissected out.

HYSTERIA

Hysteria is now comparatively rare in British dogs. Thirty-five years ago at least a dozen cases a day were treated in the clinic I attended as a student in Glasgow.

Cause

When common, hysteria was associated with the feeding of biscuits and meal pre-

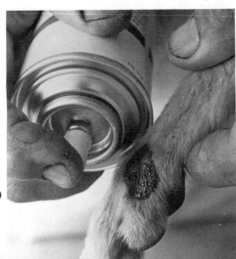

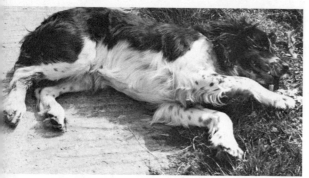

7

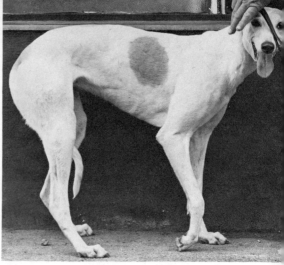

8

pared from what was called an agenised flour. This must have been a main cause because hysteria prevalence reduced spectacularly when manufacturers stopped using it.

Modern cases are attributed to a diet deficient in vitamin B_1.

I have seen the odd case apparently associated with otodectic mange.

Symptoms
A sudden noise or excitement will trigger off an attack. The dog literally 'goes mad' —racing round blindly howling its head off, oblivious to all attempts to stop it.

The attack may last for several minutes to half an hour till eventually the dog falls down in a convulsion *(photo 7)*.

Treatment
As a first-aid measure put the dog in a quiet dark room where he can do little damage—the bathroom, toilet or garage— and call your veterinary surgeon.

He will inject powerful sedative or tranquilliser, ascertain the cause, and prescribe a preventative routine.

Prevention
Change the diet. If fed mainly on biscuits, change to meat and green vegetables.

After a period of a week or two, during which tranquillisers may be necessary, the dietetical change together with a daily vitamin tablet containing vitamin B_1 should prevent further attacks.

RADIAL PARALYSIS
Cause
Injury to the radical nerve which passes round the front of the shoulder *(photo 8)*. This area is often severely bruised in accidents.

Symptoms
The elbow is markedly dropped and the dog drags the front of its toes along the ground. Sometimes the front of the carpus becomes worn raw *(photo 9)*.

Treatment
Only time can heal the injured nerve. Treatment has to be aimed at keeping the

9

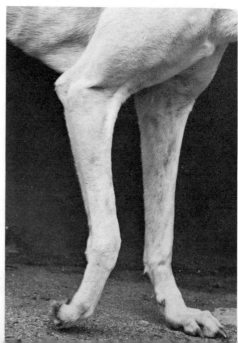

leg straight to avoid carpal or toe ulceration. Splints and plaster will probably be tried.

If the paralysis is severe and prolonged, then the leg may have to be amputated but this is a very successful operation and can be looked upon with complete confidence by the owner *(photo 10)*.

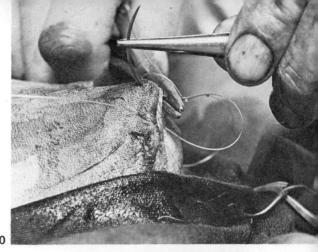

10

FACIAL PARALYSIS
Cause
Damage to the facial or trigeminal nerve which passes round the base of the ear and ramifies down the side of the face.

Symptoms
One set of jaw muscles are partially or completely paralysed, the mouth is twisted and the tongue may hang out to one side *(photo 11)*.

Treatment
Patience and time. The prognosis is quite good.

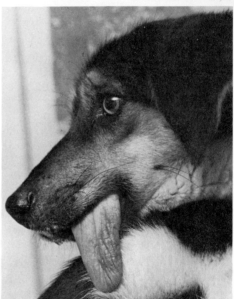

52
Poisons

OBVIOUSLY IT is not possible to deal here with all classes of poisons that are likely to affect the dog, but the following are those which occur frequently in practice.

WARFARIN POISONING

Cause
Eating rat poison which contains warfarin *(photo 1)*. Although in the small recommended quantities used in rat baits, warfarin is considered safe for pets, moderate quantities can make many a dog extremely ill or even kill it. The warfarin is an anticoagulant and produces death from internal haemorrhage.

Symptoms
Vomiting and acute depression with marked anaemia. The eye and mouth membranes are white and the inside of the mouth is ice-cold. The temperature is subnormal.

Treatment
Suspect cases should be rushed to a veterinary surgeon.

If vomiting hasn't occurred, he will vomit the dog by injecting an emetic and will inject vitamin K. If given quickly, the vitamin K will prevent internal haemorrhage. *(photo 2)*.

Where haemorrhage has occurred, recovery depends upon careful nursing. In addition to the vitamin K, the veterinary surgeon will probably prescribe vitamin B_{12} and iron.

Prevention
Don't let your pets near rat poison.

STRYCHNINE POISONING

Cause
Eating bones of vermin that have been destroyed by strychnine. Unfortunately strychnine—a vicious poison—is still avail-

1

2

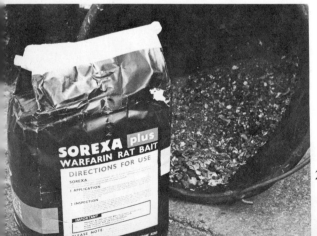

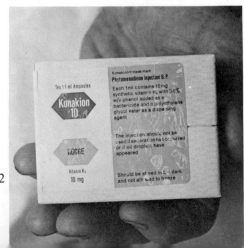

202

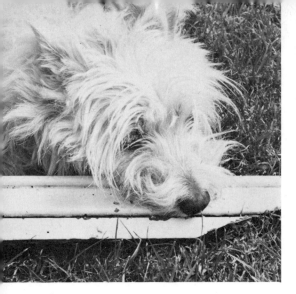

3

able to some gamekeepers. It remains in the bones of the poisoned creatures for many years.

Symptoms

Uncontrollable shaking and shivering and convulsions.

Treatment

Heavy doses of sedatives or tranquillisers. Success depends entirely on the quantity of strychnine imbibed.

LEAD POISONING

Cause

Chewing at or licking an old child's toy or a piece of wood, that has been painted with lead paint *(photo 3)*.

Symptoms

The dog slobbers at the mouth *(photo 4)*. It knuckles under at the knees, rapidly loses condition and develops chronic diarrhoea. In acute cases it will stagger about blindly and go into convulsions. Subsequently blindness can be a marked feature.

Treatment

The antidote to poisoning by lead paint is Epsom salts (magnesium sulphate) *(photo*

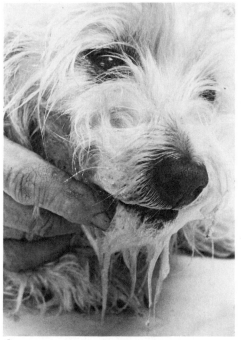

4

5). The dose is one teaspoonful twice daily of a 25 per cent solution, but it is always best to get a veterinary surgeon to make the diagnosis and prescribe the treatment.

5

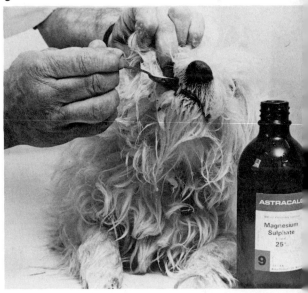

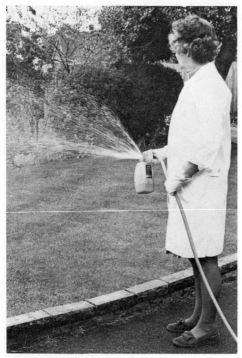

6

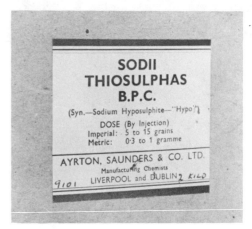

7

ARSENICAL POISONING

Cause
Licking arsenical sprays that may have been used to spray garden or farm weeds *(photo 6)*.

Symptoms
Since arsenic is an irritant poison, the symptoms are very severe, that is, those of a hypercute gastro-enteritis—severe abdominal pain with incessant vomiting which may be haemorrhagic (have blood in it). The motion is black and diarrhoeic.

If an antidote is not rapidly given, the dog will go into convulsions and die.

Treatment
The antidote is a drug called sodium thiosulphate which a veterinary surgeon will give in solution intravenously *(photo 7)*.

He will also inject tranquillisers to control the vomiting and prescribe oral demulcents—milk, kaolin etc. to allay the stomach and bowel inflammation.

It has been my experience that most cases of arsenical poisoning die.

Index